MEDICINE &
PHARMACY
IN
AMERICAN
POLITICAL
PRINTS
(1765~1870)

by William H. Helfand

American Institute of the History of Pharmacy
Madison, Wisconsin
1978

This booklet was printed through the
courtesy of
Merck Sharp & Dohme International

Publication No. 4 (New Series)
John Parascandola, General Editor
American Institute
of the History of Pharmacy
Price $10.00

The first three publications in the
Institute's new numbered series were
*Pharmacy Museums and Historical
Collections on Public View, U. S. A.*
(by Sami Hamarneh, 1972); *Historical
Hobbies for the Pharmacist* (ed. by
George Bender and John Parascandola,
1974); and *American Pharmacy in the
Colonial and Revolutionary Periods*
(ed. by George Bender and
John Parascandola, 1977).

foreword

I am profoundly indebted to the many collectors, curators and librarians, and the host of correspondents and friends who have helped me in the preparation of this book, and for their willingness to loan and give me permission to reproduce many of the illustrations which appear on the following pages.

I have acknowledged these individually, in a special section at the end of the book.

William H. Helfand

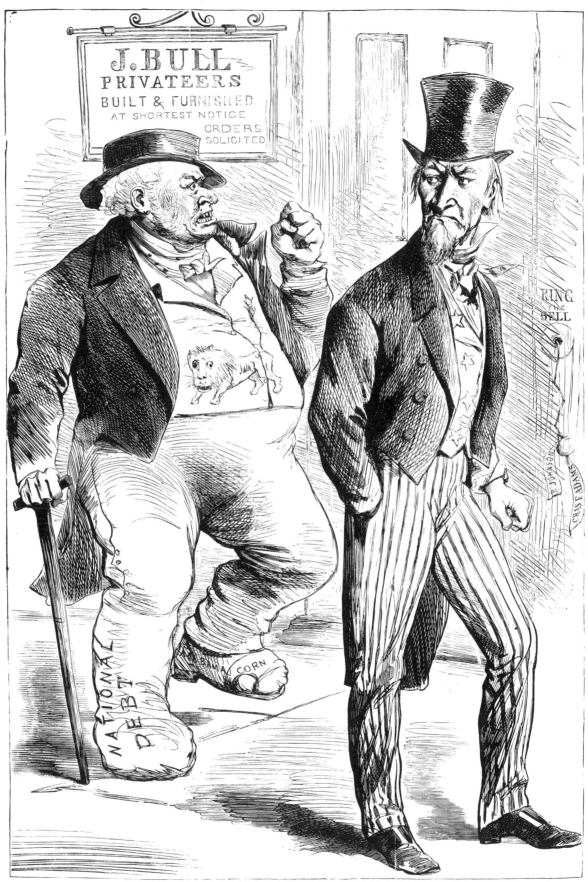

"ERROR WOUNDED WRITHES IN PAIN."

JOHN BULL. "Did you mean to step on my Corns?"
BROTHER JONATHAN. "Yes, Sir. And if you don't pay me what you ought I'll grind your Corns for you, and swell that other Foot bigger yet!"

1. "Error Wounded Writhes in Pain." Anonymous engraving, 1869. A comment on the debts owed the United States by England after the Civil War as the result of claims for Union losses due to the activities of the ship, *Alabama* (see No. 108). In the print, Brother Jonathan has stepped on John Bull's feet; each of the victim's feet is heavily bandaged, with the labels reading "Alabama Corn" and "National Debt."

From *Harper's Weekly*, Vol. 13, June 5, 1869, p. 361

introduction

In the United States the political print did not achieve significant influence until the end of the Civil War period. Then, the successful weekly humor magazines *Puck* and *Judge,* and a group of political cartoonists with insight and technical ability, including Thomas Nast, Joseph Keppler, James A. Wales and Bernhard Gillam among others, brought the art of caricature in this country to a level it had reached long before in England and France. Indeed, the thirty-year period from 1870 to 1900 in the United States has been referred to as the "golden age" of caricature.[1] Prior to this age, however, America could offer no one to rival such men as William Hogarth and James Gillray in the eighteenth century and Honoré Daumier and the Cruikshanks in the early part of the nineteenth century.

Nonetheless, the political print in the United States was a frequently used vehicle for the expression of opinion during the nation's first hundred years. Approximately one thousand political caricatures were published as separate prints in the period up to 1870,[2] and this number is more than doubled if the cartoons in the weekly and monthly journals that began to appear in the 1840's are included. With the advent of cheaper and more efficient lithographic processes, the individual print, issued as a separate, almost ceased as an entity by 1870; its place was taken by the cartoons in many weekly and a few daily newspapers. Today's newspaper cartoons are the potent descendants of this tradition of political caricature, but there are now only a few weekly or monthly journals that print cartoons regularly.

These caricatures have long been familiar to those interested in the history of medicine and pharmacy who have used them as illuminating source material in the study of social and political history; they can be used as a source of metaphors and references to illustrate the problems of contemporary life. Looked at in this way, the caricatures produced in the first half of the nineteenth century, and in the years before the institutionalization of cartoons in the daily and weekly press, provide a setting for a variety of political attitudes. In many cases, the setting is a medical one, for medicine was such an important part of social life, a medical theme could also be used as background, for quick understanding, in conveying attitudes toward political questions. Since the objective of the artist was in almost every case propaganda, the setting of his illustration had to evoke immediate recognition in the mind of the viewer; medicine, illness, prescriptions, the sick bed, nursing, etc., were parts of everyday life, and it is therefore not surprising that they were used with some frequency by the cartoonist. In some prints, the medical or pharmaceutical reference is incidental to the general theme of the print in question; in others, it is more intimately related.

When considering such material, the British and French efforts come to mind immediately; American political caricatures are less well-known, but exist nonetheless, and it is the purpose of this study to examine some examples of this American production. If we use the year 1870 as a cutoff point in considering those political prints that have some relevance to medicine and pharmacy, there are more than a hundred items that can be included. Roughly half of these are individual prints (mostly before the Civil War) and the rest are from serial publications. There are also several examples used as propaganda on the envelopes produced on a large scale during the Civil War period.

classification

The broad areas covered by these illustrations which sought to provide almost instant recall and association relate to the physician's tasks of diagnosis and examination, to types of illness, to medical procedures, to systems of medicine, to drugs and pharmacy, and to the administration of medicines. Under each of these headings there are, of course, variations, but not surprisingly, many of the same themes appear more than once. Nor were such themes peculiar to the early social history of this country; they can be found in earlier British, French, and German prints and in modern twentieth century cartoons as well. There is even some evidence that "all the real, solid, elemental jests against doctors were uttered some one or two thousand years ago."[3]

The prints that have medical interest have been grouped into the categories noted above. They include, in addition to those of direct political relevance, a number of examples that comment on aspects of the Civil War which are only political because they relate to the war. Some showing soldiers in a medical setting or street scenes before a drug store have been included because they were created to illustrate an event of political importance. That the medical portion of the print was of no direct importance to the event itself is certainly true; the same can be said of many of the caricatures. Perhaps the only group of pictures not included, that might be considered to fall into the same category as these Civil War scenes, is the illustrations of hospitals, but there are a sufficient number of these to warrant separate treatment. The prints with medical or pharmaceutical significance are illustrated with brief notes throughout the text. A chronological list appears on page 80. Where possible, bibliographic references to each of the prints are given, and a composite bibliography of these references can be found on page 83.

The following sections summarize the content and character of the prints in accordance with the categories noted above. The numbers in each instance refer to the checklist.

1. Roger Butterfield, *The American Past,*
   Simon & Schuster, New York, 1947, p. 291
2. William Murrell, *A History of American Graphic Humor,*
   Whitney Museum of American Art, New York, NY, 1933, Vol. I, p. 116
3. Charles L. Dana, "The Evil Spoken of Physicians,"
   Proc. Charaka Club, 1902, I. p. 80

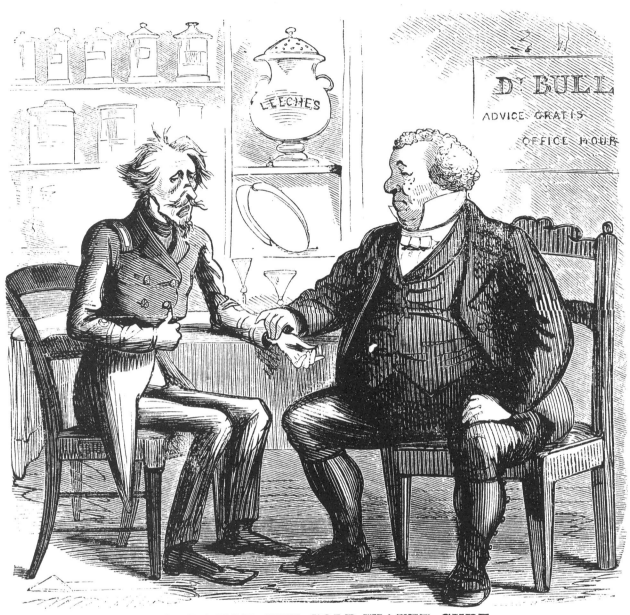

A CASE FOR THE COLD-WATER CURE.

DOCTOR BULL. "Are you subject to these attacks?"

CAPTAIN SEMMES. "No, DOCTOR; this is the first of the kind. The fact is, heretofore I have been very careful to avoid exposure to any thing which might produce the slightest reaction."

DOCTOR BULL. "But, about this affair; how did it come on?"

CAPTAIN SEMMES. "Well, first I experienced a sort of Shooting in the Side, accompanied by Symptoms of Collapse, followed by a General Sinking, and a kind of Swimming Sensation."

DOCTOR BULL. "Yes, yes — exactly! I think I had slight symptoms of the disorder myself some years ago. It is known among the profession as *Yankeephobia*, for which Spirit of Cave-in is frequently used: but in your case, I should recommend building up—a little iron, and so forth. However, I will fix you up something which will make a man of you in no time."

2. A Case for the Cold-Water Cure. Engraving by Frank Bellew, 1864.
Britain, as a supporter of the South through the war years, came in for its share
of satirical treatment. This cartoon shows Dr. Bull taking the pulse of his patient;
in the background are jars of drugs and one for leeches.

From *Harper's Weekly*, Vol. 8, July 23, 1864, p. 480

establishing a diagnosis

The examination of a patient in order to diagnose his ailments was a subject used often in this series of American prints. Of course, the theme lent itself to political caricature, for a diagnosis can be of a political situation as well as of a specific patient's condition. The physician's search for a proper diagnosis involves the quest for a definitive understanding, and in the political cartoons where the theme was used, the artist frequently would show a physician examining a patient to identify what was considered to be the political "illness" causing the problem. *A Case for the Cold-Water Cure* can serve as a typical example: here the physician is Britain, as personified by "Doctor" John Bull, shown taking the pulse of his distressed patient, Raphael Semmes (No. 2). As the captain of the Confederate warship, the *Alabama*, Semmes had caused great damage to Union merchant shipping from the beginning of his operations in 1862 until his ship was sunk in 1864 (the "cold water" noted in the title). Throughout the war Britain had hedged its neutrality by selling arms and goods to both sides although it tended to sympathize with the Confederacy for economic reasons. As pointed out in the print, Britain's "prescription" for the destroyed *Alabama* and the "Yankeephobia" of its captain was ironclad ships, the "iron" Dr. Bull recommends. The release of these ironclad "Laird rams" to the Confederacy, for whom they were being made and fitted, would have proven a disastrous blow to the Union. They might well have become a *causus belli* between the Union and Great Britain had not the British government finally seized them in October, 1863 rather than permit their release to the Confederacy.

Both the South and the North appeared as patients in several of the prints issued during the Civil War, but other political events made use of the same concept. During the 1840's, the Locofoco faction of the Democratic Party (a radical, urban wing of supporters of Jacksonian democracy), was the subject of constant attacks by the press. The decline and demise of the Locofocos, so ardently desired by their adversaries, were almost gleefully portrayed in two caricatures of the period that show an animal as the symbol of the group; in one case the patient is dying and in the second has succumbed and is being subjected to a coroner's inquest (Nos. 3 and 4). In other prints the theme of a

3. The death of Locofocoism. Anonymous lithograph, 1840.
A satire on the Loco-foco Democrats and their alliance with the Jackson-Van Buren party. The patient has horns and is attended by seven physicians. Among them is Calhoun, who holds a bottle of "Calhoun's Locofoco Life Preserver." and there are other medicines on a table, including "Dr. Dungan's Soporific." "Benton Drops," "Treasury Pap," and "Poinsetts Indian Pills." Jackson is depicted as the wife of the dying patient. Calhoun complains of the loss of not only Locofocoism, but also his "last patient Nullification," and is afraid he "must *once* more change my system or give up practice."

Weitenkampf, p. 65

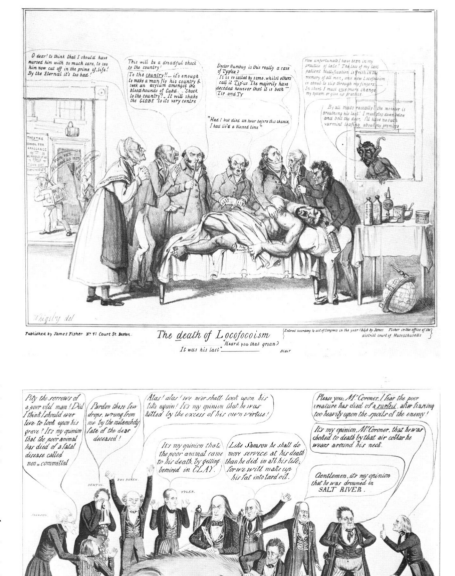

The death of Locofocoism

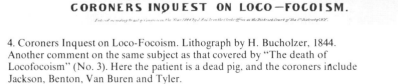

CORONERS INQUEST ON LOCO—FOCOISM.

4. Coroners Inquest on Loco-Focoism. Lithograph by H. Bucholzer, 1844.
Another comment on the same subject as that covered by "The death of Locofocoism" (No. 3). Here the patient is a dead pig, and the coroners include Jackson, Benton, Van Buren and Tyler.

Weitenkampf, p. 83

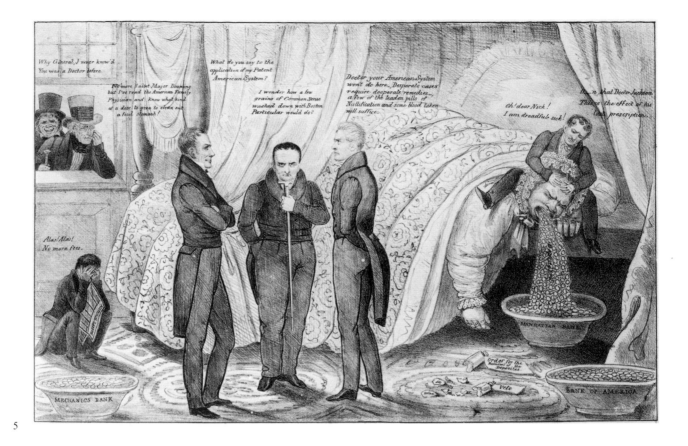

5

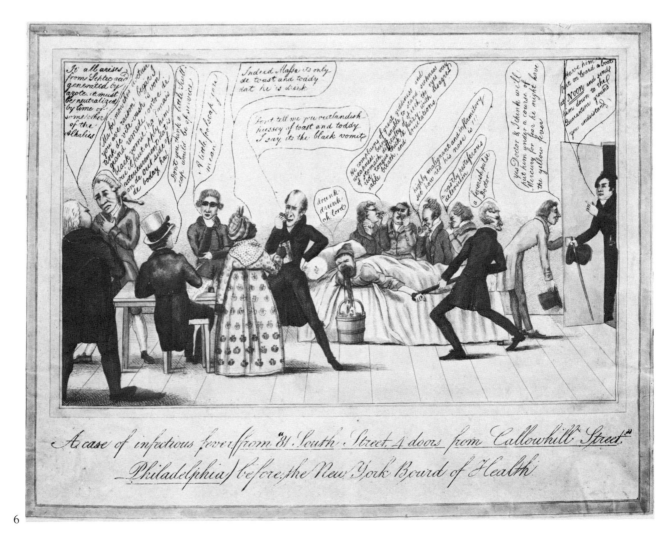

6

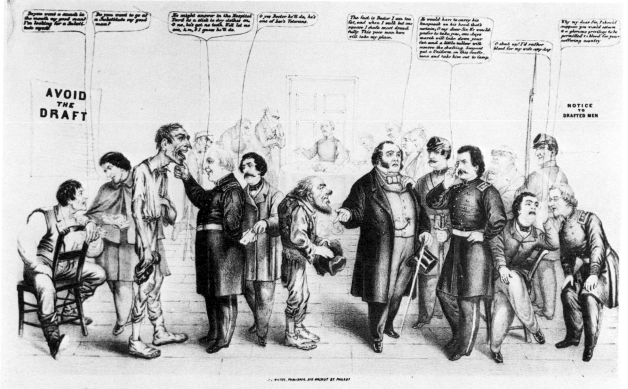

OFFERING A SUBSTITUTE. A SCENE IN THE OFFICE OF THE PROVOST MARSHALL.

7

5. The Doctors Puzzled or the Desperate
Case of Mother U.S. Bank.
Anonymous lithograph, c. 1833.
Another print on the controversy over the
national bank. The patient, in bed, vomits
"Deposites." Nicholas Biddle, then President
of the Bank, holding her, says "D___n that
Doctor Jackson. This is the effect of his last
prescription." On the floor lie broken bottles
of "Veto" and "Order for the Removal of the
Deposites." The two figures at the window
are Andrew Jackson and Major Downing.
The three doctors holding a consultation are
Clay, Webster and Calhoun. There is also a
physician present complaining "Alas! Alas!
No more fees."

Weitenkampf, p. 28; Butterfield, p. 91;
Vinson, p. 51; Hess & Kaplan, pp. 66-67

6. A case of infectious fever,
(from "81 South Street, 4 doors from
Callowhill Street," Philadelphia) before
the New York Board of Health.
Anonymous engraving, 1820.
A print illustrating attitudes toward
appointed Public Health officials in two large
cities, Philadelphia and New York. A series
of New York physicians are shown discussing
the case of a sick patient on a couch but are
less able to diagnose the true problem—
drunkenness—than a black woman who is
also present. Several of them comment on the
remedy for the illness.

Murrell I, p. 99; Weitenkampf, p. 20

7. Offering a Substitute. A Scene in the
Office of the Provost Marshall.
Anonymous lithograph, 1862.
The subject of this print is the Civil War
draft, and depicts the examination of
prospective soldiers. Two physicians, one of
whom is taking a bribe, are shown examining
the candidates.

Weitenkampf, p. 135

patient being treated is picked up in commentaries on the financial
problems of the nation (No. 5) and, on a local level, indicating both the
local rivalry and the parlous state of medicine in the early nineteenth
century in an illustration of several New York doctors attempting to
analyze the cause of *A case of infectious fever* which had been con-
tracted in Philadelphia (No. 6).

The subject of establishing a diagnosis also was particularly adapt-
able to offering a commentary on military conscription, a subject discussed frequently during the years of the Civil War. The setting up of
the draft was something new and alien to the American consciousness,
and views on it, both pro and con, appeared with some frequency in
newspapers and journals. Naturally, there were many men who resisted
the thought of going into battle for even the noblest of causes. Out of
this fear of military service sprang corruption. A man, once drafted, was
able to "buy" someone as his replacement for a price that usually aver-
aged around $300. The substitute has to be "fit for duty," a subjective
term open to interpretation. In the print entitled *Offering a Substitute.
A Scene in the Office of the Provost Marshall,* published in 1862, two
physicians are shown examining some prospective draft choices (No. 7).
One of them studies the teeth of the proposed substitute, a human
wreck who, he decides, is fit for service at the very moment he feels
money in his palm. In contrast, a well-dressed prospect with some legitimate medical complaints is doomed for military service. His would-
be substitute, a hunchbacked dwarf, is justifiably rejected if only because the specific consideration needed to ensure his enlistment had not
been proffered.

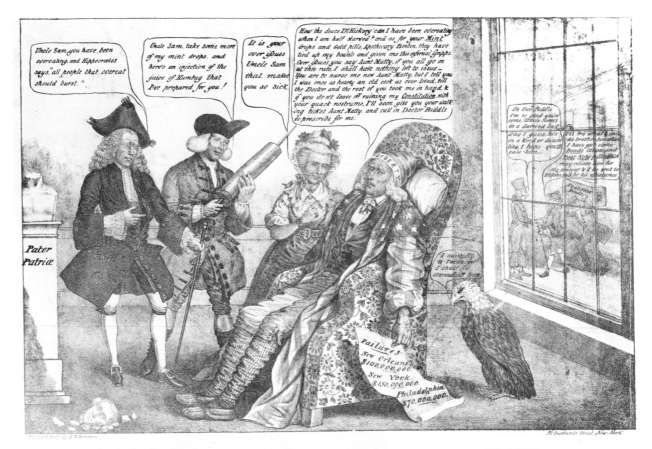

UNCLE SAM SICK WITH LA GRIPPE.

8

TROUBLED TREASURES

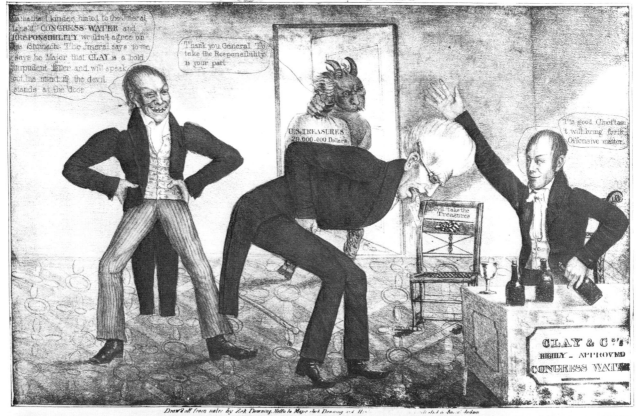

9

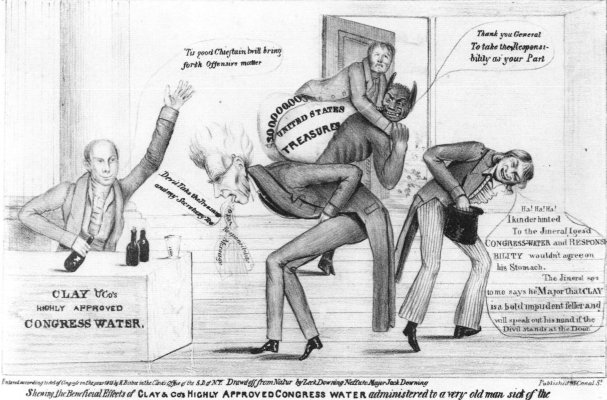

Shewing the Beneficial Effects of CLAY & Co's HIGHLY APPROVED CONGRESS WATER administered to a very old man sick of the
Deposite Fever caused by wearing VAN BUREN'S newly invented Patent Magic High Pressure Cabinet Spectacles

10

illnesses

The prints in the category of "Illnesses" show a variety of medical conditions, both real and imaginary. The former include the common cold, gout, fainting, toothache, cholera, typhus, lockjaw, tapeworms and trouble with corns, while the fictional ones add to the medical lexicon such novelties as the "Oregon Fever," "Chronophobia," "Tip-us" and "Confederate Rash." But even though illnesses of all sorts afflicted the body politic, those of most frequency appeared to attack the gut and the respiratory tract. Sniffling, sneezing, vomiting and diarrhea were often used by American caricaturists to illustrate some internal political malaise or the effects of events that were politically contentious.

An 1838 lithograph by H. R. Robinson, *Uncle Sam Sick with La Grippe*, uses these themes most effectively (No. 8). The financial panic of 1837 was brought about by what many critics believed to be outright blundering on the part of the Democratic party. President Jackson, in 1836, had issued a notice to government land agents that only specie and no paper bank notes would be accepted as payment for federal lands. The country at the time was expanding exponentially and Jackson's Specie Circular soon helped deplete the banks of whatever hard money was on hand. With the number of bank failures mounting rapidly, Jackson notes that Uncle Sam has been overeating, but the patient asks, "How the deuce Dr. Hickory can I have been overeating when I'm half starved." The doctor attending Uncle Sam is Andrew Jackson (Old Hickory), and his supporter, Senator Thomas Hart Benton of Missouri, is shown as the apothecary, carrying an oversized clyster as his symbol of office. The nurse in the print is still another member of the Democratic leadership, Martin Van Buren, who had assumed the presidency just before the panic of 1837 broke. The attempts of the three to cure the patient of overeating have produced the double-barreled effect of

8. Uncle Sam Sick with La Grippe.
Lithograph by H.R. Robinson, 1838.
This print discusses the economic problems affecting the United States after the Panic of 1837. It shows the patient, Uncle Sam, treated by several people, including Jackson, Benton and Van Buren. Benton, the apothecary, holds a clyster. Outside the patient's room, Dr. Biddle is being greeted warmly by Brother Jonathan, making this the earliest print, and one of the few ever made, in which both Uncle Sam and Brother Jonathan appear.

Murrell I, pp. 131-133; Weitenkampf, p. 36

9. Troubled Treasures.
Lithograph by E. Bisbee, 1833.
One of the many prints relating to the efforts of Andrew Jackson to do away with the Bank of the United States by refusing to renew its charter. Here Jackson is vomiting "Veto," "Responsibility," "Message," while Henry Clay sells the possible cause of his distress, "Clay & Co's Highly Approved Congress Water." Major Jack Downing, an individual who appears in many of the contemporary satirical prints, looks on.

Weitenkampf, p. 29.

10. Troubled Treasures.
Lithograph by R. Bisbee, 1833.
This print is similar to No. 9, but is more crudely drawn, and the figures are reversed.

Weitenkampf, p. 29

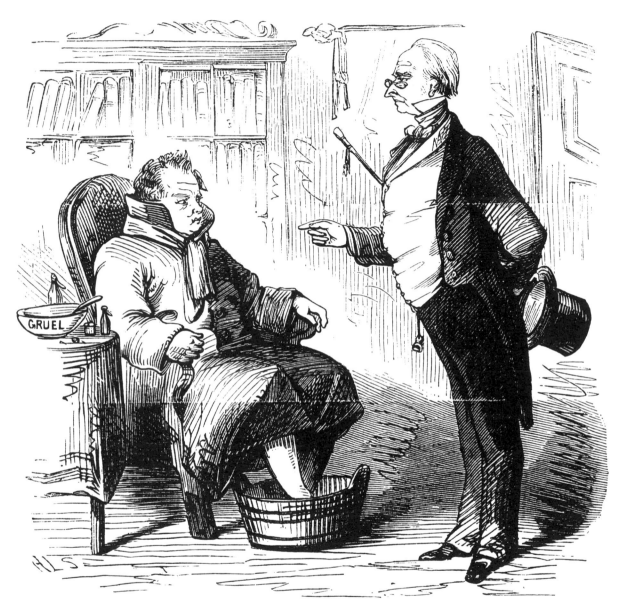

THE POLITICAL INVALID..

S. A. Douglas.—Do you think I'm a very sick man, Doctor?

Doctor Jonathan.—Yes, Stephen; the Charleston air disagreed with you decidedly, and I'm very much afraid that that of Baltimore wont be much better.

11. The Political Invalid. Engraving by H. L. Stevens, 1860.
A satire on Stephen Douglas, one of the candidates running against Lincoln in the election of 1860. He is shown as a sick patient, his feet in a bucket, talking to Dr. Jonathan. Some of his medicines are nearby.

From *Vanity Fair*, Vol. 1, June 16, 1860, p. 387; Shaw, p. 77

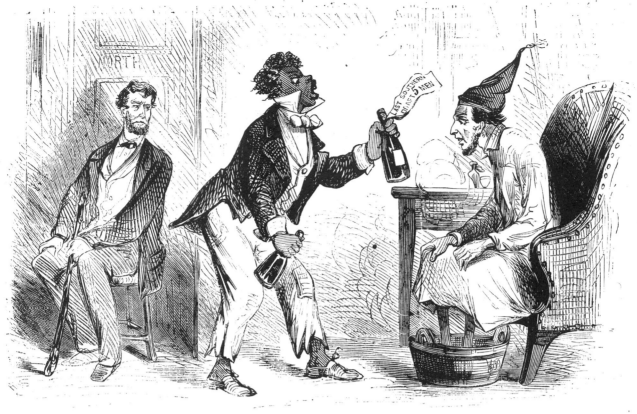

THAT DRAFT.

JEFF DAVIS. "Shut the Door, SLIDELL ALEXANDER, I'm shivering all over! That Draft from the North will be the death of me — *I feel it!*"

SLIDELL ALEXANDER. "C-c-cant shut it, Massa. ABE LINCOLN's *got his Back 'gainst it.* Better try a little 'o dis de Doctor left yer."

12. That Draft. Anonymous engraving, 1862.
Another comment on the draft. This print shows Jefferson Davis,
his feet in a tub of hot water, offered medicine labeled
"Last Southern Draft 5 Men." Lincoln looks on quietly.

From *Harper's Weekly*, Vol. 6, Oct. 4, 1862, p. 640; Wilson, p. 183

tying up the patient's bowels and giving him the grippe. To recover, Uncle Sam has to call in Doctor Biddle (Nicholas Biddle had been President of the United States Bank) in his attempt to return to the more conservative and centralized banking system which the Bank of the United States represented. The print is most effective in making use of several medical themes to criticize the fiscal programs of the Jackson administration. It is also the first published print to use two familiar symbols of the nation, Uncle Sam and Brother Jonathan, in the same illustration. And it also gives us one of the rare American uses of the clyster, an instrument which figures so prominently in the French political prints of the eighteenth and nineteenth centuries.[4]

Biddle's Bank of the United States earlier had seemed to provoke a minor epidemic of gastrointestinal complaints. In *Troubled Treasures*, a cartoon published in 1833, Andrew Jackson is taken to task for his failure to renew the Bank's charter (Nos. 9 and 10). Henry Clay had made the Bank a campaign issue in 1832. Andrew Jackson swallowed the challenge whole, so to speak, and the effect of his taking Clay's "highly approved" panacea was to cause him to vomit "offensive matter." This "matter" consisted of his

vetoing the re-chartering of the Bank, a veto "message" that attacked big banking interests, and his promise of government "responsibility" for the financial well-being of the common people. With Jackson thus engaged, the devil is able to leave with both the federal deposits and the Secretary of the Treasury in his possession. In the print, the transfer of funds from the stable Bank of the United States to the uncertain, unproven local banks is implied. One additional commentator shown on the right in the print is Major Jack Downing, the personification of the interests of the common man; he is a recurring figure in the political cartoons of the period.

The caricatures using the common cold or influenza usually show the patients either slumped in a chair or with their feet in buckets of hot water, with the physician looking on. Both Stephen Douglas, Lincoln's opponent in the election of 1860, and Jefferson Davis, the head of the Confederacy during the Civil War, are given this treatment in the prints (Nos. 11 and 12).

4. W. H. Helfand, "Medicine and Pharmacy in French Political Prints," *Transactions and Studies of the College of Physicians of Philadelphia*, 4th Ser., 1974, 42, I, July, p. 17

13

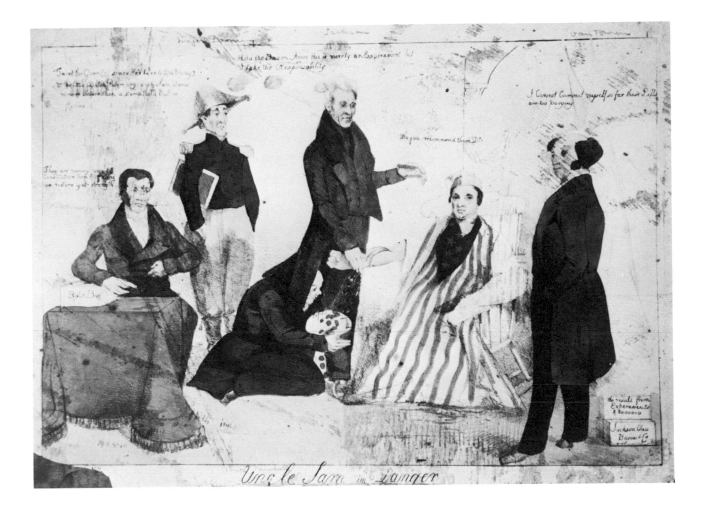

Uncle Sam in Danger

medical procedures

Bleeding the patient was a widely accepted therapeutic procedure in the eighteenth and nineteenth centuries, and provided the artist with a favorite device as sharp as the doctor's lancet. As a rule, it was used to illustrate some financial problem, either the difficulties of the state, or the heavy taxation of individuals. There are several examples, but one of the anti-Jacksonian cartoons, *Uncle Sam in Danger*, provides a typical example (No. 13). Again, the bank policy of the government is the theme and the bleeding of Uncle Sam is apparently in reference to the federal funds transferred from the Bank of the United States to a number of local banks. Whig opposition was frightened by the prospect of the funneling of money into "pet banks" of the Democrats where, they alleged, credit policies favored those who voted the Democratic ticket. Jackson is shown letting blood into a basin held by one of his close advisors, Amos Kendall. Major Downing describes his pessimism about this method of "cure" when he says "Twixt the Gimril [Jackson]… and the little Dutch Potercary [Van Buren] Uncle Sam stands no more chance than a stump tail'd Bull in fly time." Another onlooker suggests the ingestion of ballots (an election) as a cure, but Van Buren criticizes this as being "too purging." But Van Buren, as it turned out, had little to worry about for he assumed the Presidency in 1837, three years after the print was issued.

Surgery was another procedure shown in the prints, in one case with Van Buren as the patient and in another with Lincoln about to perform an operation on Siamese twins, with James Buchanan and James Gordon Bennett, two of his political opponents, replacing the famous Chang and Eng (Nos. 14 and 15).

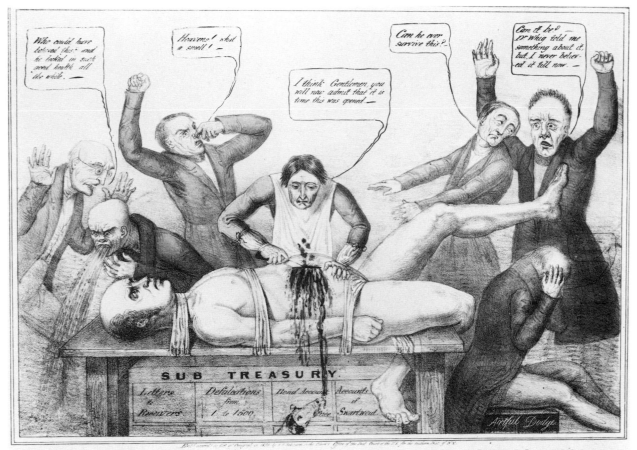

PROFESSOR WISE, Performing a Surgical Operation in CONGRESS HALL.

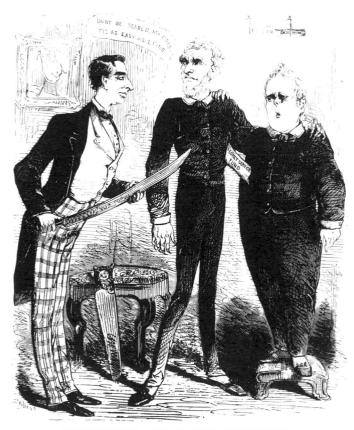

WONDERFUL SURGICAL OPERATION,
PERFORMED BY DOCT. LINCOLN ON THE POLITICAL CHANG AND ENG.
POLITICAL CHANG, J. B———N.
POLITICAL ENG, J. G. B———T.

14. Professor Wise, Performing a Surgical
Operation in Congress Hall.
Lithograph by H. R. Robinson, 1839.
A print commenting on the financial
problems plaguing the Van Buren
administration. The surgeon is Henry
Alexander Wise, a member of Congress from
Virginia, one of Van Buren's opponents, who
notes, "I think Gentlemen, you will now
admit that it is time this was opened," as he
operates on a bloody Van Buren. The
onlookers are all sickened by the odor and
perhaps the nature of the operation itself.

Weitenkampf, p. 57

15. Wonderful Surgical Operation.
Engraving by H. L. Stephens, 1860.
Buchanan, the retiring president, and
Bennett, the editor, both opposed Lincoln's
candidacy. In this print Lincoln is a surgeon,
about to operate on the Siamese twins,
Buchanan and Bennett.

From *Vanity Fair*, Vol. 2, Nov. 3, 1860,
p. 225, Wilson, p. 73; Shaw, p. 143

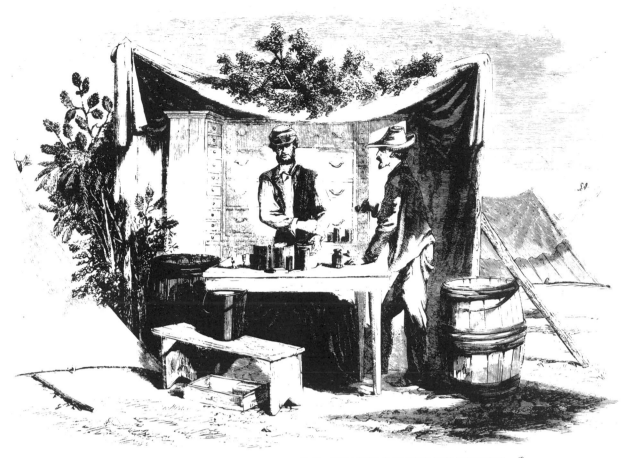

CAMP SCENES—AN ARMY DRUG STORE—THE HOSPITAL STEWARD.—FROM A SKETCH BY OUR SPECIAL ARTIST, JOSEPH BECKER.

16

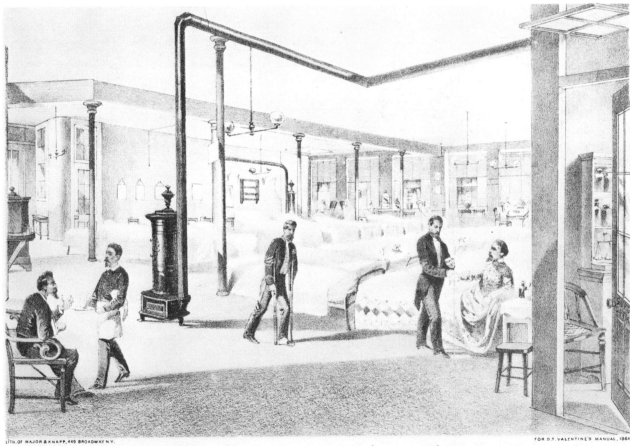

SOLDIER'S DEPOT, HOSPITAL (4TH FLOOR)

17

16. Camp Scenes—An Army Drug Store—The Hospital Steward.
Engraving after Joseph Becker, 1864.
A field pharmacy during the Civil War. A pharmacist is shown
at a table on which are some medicines, and in the rear are
cabinets for additional medicines.

From *Frank Leslie's Illustrated Newspaper*, Vol. 19, Nov. 12,
1864, p. 117, G. W. Smith, *Medicines for the Union Army*,
Madison, 1962, Title Page

17. Soldier's Depot, Hospital (4th floor).
Lithograph by Major and Knapp, 1864.
A view of the interior of a hospital in which soldiers are
recuperating from injuries sustained in the fighting. A physician
takes the pulse of one; another walks on crutches. At one side part
of the interior of the hospital pharmacy can be seen.

From *Valentine's Manual*, New York, 1864

18. To The Surgeon. Anonymous Comic Valentine, c. 1861.
A satire on the surgeons attending the troops during the Civil War.
A skeleton is shown carrying surgical instruments which include
a large saw.

Dannett, p. 178

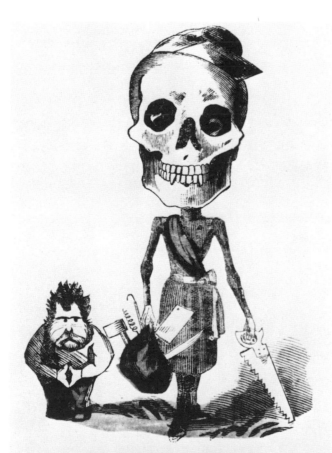

TO THE SURGEON.

Ho! ho! old saw bones, here you come,
Yes, when the rebels whack us.
You are always ready with your traps,
To mangle. saw, and hack us.

The Civil War took a heavy toll of human life, a significant proportion of which was due to the inadequacies of medical techniques and facilities behind the front lines. Available figures indicate that almost twice as many Union soldiers died from disease as from wounds received in battle. Antisepsis was, of course, not practiced and anesthetics were not always available.

Hospitals were usually improvised affairs manned by a few overworked doctors and care was often less than ideal (Nos. 16 and 17). Abdominal wounds or major amputations meant almost certain death. One attitude towards the fear of surgical procedures is given in a comic valentine published during the war, the verse of which reads,

Ho! ho! old saw bones, here you come,
Yes, when the rebels whack us,
You are always ready with your traps,
To mangle, saw, and hack us (No. 18)

In addition to bleeding and surgery, the prints show other procedures in use during the period. These include the administration of enemas, amputation, autopsy and dentistry. In choosing these themes, American artists were no different than their counterparts in France and England, for subjects such as bleeding, cutting off a limb, extracting a tooth, and giving a clyster, are all excellent vehicles for offering opinions about the evils and excesses of politics and the state. And, not surprisingly, these themes are still in frequent use today.

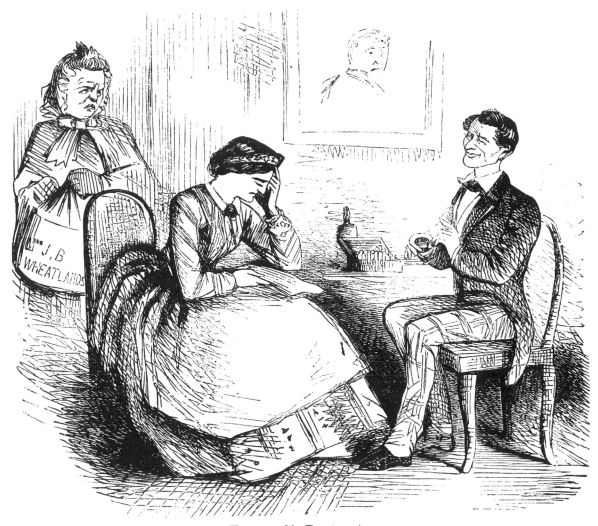

Homeopathic Treatment.
Vide *Herald*, Feb. 11th, p. 4.

Dr. Lincoln (to Miss Columbia).—Now, MISS COLUMBIA, IF YOU WILL FOLLOW MY PRESCRIPTIONS, WHICH ARE OF AN EXTREMELY MILD CHARACTER, BUT WHICH YOUR OLD NURSE, MRS. BUCHANAN, SEEMS TO HAVE BEEN SO AVERSE TO, I HAVE NO DOUBT BUT THAT THE UNION WILL BE RESTORED TO POSITION, HEALTH, AND VIGOR.

19. Homeopathic Treatment. Anonymous engraving, 1861.
A print illustrating Lincoln's approach to the problems of maintaining the integrity of the Union, after inheriting them from Buchanan. Lincoln is the doctor, advising the patient, Columbia, to follow his prescriptions. Buchanan looks on grimly, but Lincoln, his box of homeopathic pills beside him, looks most confident.

From *Yankee Notions*, Vol. 10, April, 1861, p. 109; Shaw, p. 225; Wilson, p. 121

systems of medicine

Although most of the prints with a medical subject show medicine as practiced in an orthodox manner, there are a few presenting alternative approaches. In a print issued in 1861 Lincoln is shown as a homeopath treating Columbia, a distraught frowning patient, with his prescriptions, some of which can be seen in a box the doctor has brought along (No. 19). The patient, representing the Union, has been taken ill by the turmoil of 1861. Lincoln has just assumed office, and the shadowy caricature of James Buchanan, the former President, can be seen slipping out the door. Buchanan had confronted the issue of Southern secession timidly and when Lincoln took office the problem

needed immediate treatment. Lincoln refused to accept secession and took steps to supply the beleaguered Fort Sumter. Thus, Lincoln's bold position is satirized by the cartoonist as a homeopathic cure "…my prescriptions, which are of an extremely mild character…." One month later Miss Columbia's "disease" came to a head and the Civil War began.

Phrenology had been a well-known system of diagnosis in the United States as a result of its popularization by Johann Christoph Spurzheim and Orson Fowler, and it was the subject of several prints. In one, Columbia is again the patient, and in another, Zachary Taylor is shown being examined in the New York

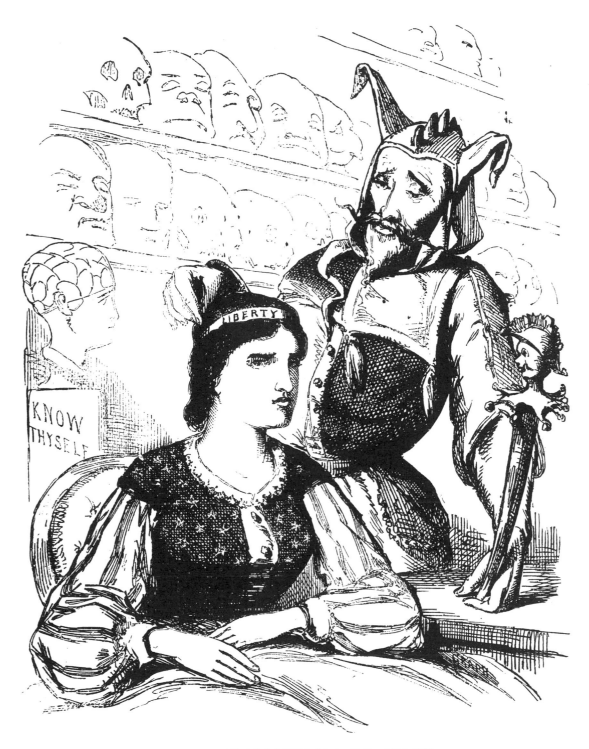

OUR BIOLOGO-MEDICO-PHRENOLOGY.

VANITY FAIR.—" *My dear Miss Union, your symptoms are very alarming. Naturally of a sanguine-nervous temperament, irritation has rendered you bilious, while the phlebotomy to which you have been recklessly subjected is rapidly reducing you to a lymphatic state. The condition of your mind justifies me in saying that you must abandon homœopathic practice and give up milk-and-water diet. Plenty of Iron, with no end of Draughts, is what you require. Your fortitude, your patience, under bad treatment, has indeed been beyond praise ; but, unless your physicians pay more regard to your Constitution, I cannot be answerable for your life. You should insist upon knowing what their prescriptions mean before you pay their bills. Then with action, vigorous action, your health will be speedily restored.*"

20. Our Biologo-Medico-Phrenology. Anonymous engraving, 1862.
The problems besetting the Union are analyzed by a phrenologist in this print, with not only diagnosis, but also the prescribed course of therapy being fully discussed in the caption.

From *Vanity Fair*, Vol. 6, Oct. 4, 1862, p. 162

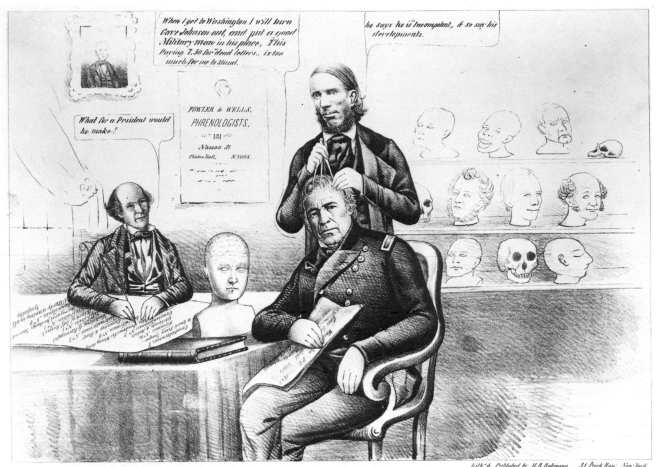

When I get to Washington I will turn Cave Johnson out, and put a good Military man in his place, This Paying 7.50 for dead letters.. is too much for me to stand.

he says he is "Incompetent,, & so say his developments.

What for a President would he make!

FOWLER & WELLS.
PHRENOLOGISTS.
131
Nassau St.
Clinton Hall,   N. YORK.

THE CANDIDATE OF MANY PARTIES.

A Phrenological Examination to Ascertain What His Political Principles Are.

Lith'd & Published by H. R. Robinson   31 Park Row New York

21. The Candidate of Many Parties. Lithograph by H. R. Robinson, 1848.
A satire on the qualifications for the presidency of one of the candidates, Zachary Taylor. The print shows him undergoing
a phrenological examination in the offices of Fowler and Wells.

Weitenkampf, p. 93

offices of Fowler and Wells (Nos. 20 and 21). In the latter, *The Candidate of Many Parties*, the purpose of the artist was to present some opinions on Taylor after he had been nominated as the Whig party candidate at their convention in Philadelphia. His opponents in the election of 1848 were Lewis Cass and Martin Van Buren, and Taylor, the eventual victor, had been relatively unknown to most of the nation prior to his nomination. Taylor had recently served as a general in the Mexican War–he was known as the "hero of Buena Vista,"–and his military successes had earned him considerable popularity. Although he lacked political experience the Whig party selected him in their eagerness for a winning candidate. In many quarters there was great doubt about his competence to lead the nation. So obscure was Taylor's political position that the artist felt it advisable to show him being scruti-

nized by phrenologists, who hoped to uncover his politics by interpreting the bumps on his head.

Quackery in general has always afforded a proper subject with which to attack any political figure who needed to be criticized, and several prints of the period refer to quacks and charlatans. In one of these, *Confab between John Bull and Brother Jonathan*, the latter has had to have his leg amputated because he had accepted the advice of quacks in the treatment of his corns (No. 22). As a result, his parting advice to John Bull is "...whatever you do, never suffer yourself to be operated upon by quacks; however plausible they may talk, they'll ruin your Constitution, and not leave you a leg to stand upon." The barb was directed against the economic difficulties that followed Jackson's financial policies.

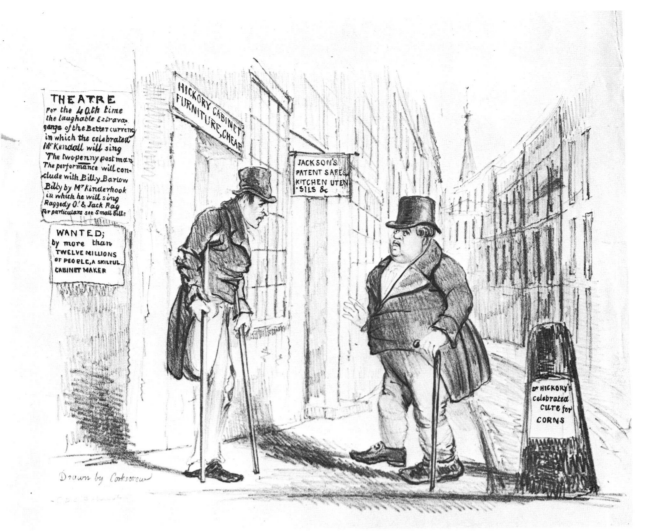

CONFAB BETWEEN JOHN BULL AND BROTHER JONATHAN.

J. Bull.—Why, brother Jonathan, 'ow 'orrid hunwell you do look! What his the matter? Lost a leg, too! Well, I 'eard you was a little lame, but I'd no idea it was any think so bad.

B. Jonathan.—Ah, brother John, thereby hangs a tale. Some time ago, I had a corn on my great toe; I did 'nt mind it much, though it twinged a little now and then, when trod upon, or when I was thoughtless enough to put on a tight shoe. Howsomever, some of my folks said I ought to look to it in time, so I submitted it to the examination of Dr. Hickory, Dr. Kinderhook, and a few other celebrated doctors of this class—all rank quacks, between you and I, as ever lived;—unluckily I did n't know it at the time.—Well, the result of the examination was, that my whole system would shortly be affected, and nothing but amputation could save me. So I suffered the limb to be lopped off, like a fool, instead of following the advice of several regularly graduated physicians, who asserted that a little rasping and corn plaster would be quite sufficient to effect a cure.

J. Bull.—My hye! Why, brother Jonathan, what a judy you must a' been. I would 't apply such a remedy to cure the gout that I've 'ad hall my life.

B. Jonathan.—Oh, brother John, I would 'nt have suffered the operation, had not one of the quacks who was *bent on* amputation assured me that he had discovered a *specie*-fic, that would not only heal the stump immediately, but would cause a sound leg to grow out in two or three weeks. Alas! it's now upwards of twelve months, and I can hardly hobble about. I have not been able to earn any thing since; I am going to *rags*. By the bye, I owe you a little change. I have 'nt it about me just now.

J. Bull.—Well, that's unlucky, brother Jonathan, as I have several notes to pay, and am much in want of money; at the same time I am sorry to see you so unfortunate and so down at the 'eel. To think that a man at your time of life should have one foot in the grave! it's mortifying.

B. Jonathan.—Oh, I don't care how much that is mortifying; the worst of it is, my rascally operators are now apprehensive of mortification in the stump they have left me; should this be the case, I shall soon have two feet in the grave. Oh, brother John! brother John! whatever you do, never suffer yourself to be operated upon by quacks; however plausible they may talk, they'll ruin your CONSTITUTION, and not leave you a leg to stand upon.

22. Confab between John Bull and Brother Jonathan. Lithograph by D. C. Johnston, 1836.
The economic problems resulting from Jackson's veto of the Bank charter are the subject of this caricature. A one-legged Brother Jonathan on crutches, discusses his problems with John Bull. A sign advertises "Dr. Hickory's Celebrated Cure for Corns." Jonathan comments that he had submitted his corns to examination by certain quacks, with drastic results.

Weitenkampf, p. 40

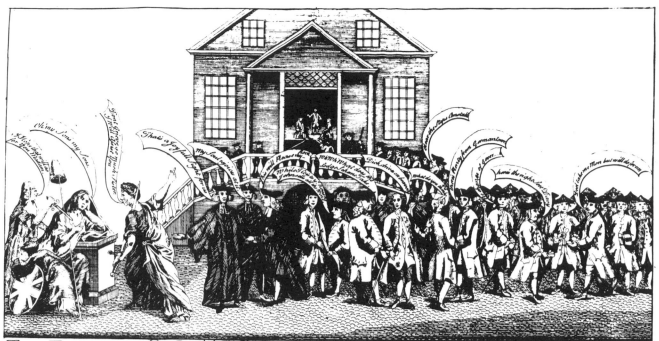

THE ELECTION *Humbly Inscrib'd, to the Saturday-Nights Club, in Lodge Alley.*
Calm thinking Villains whom no faith can fix, Of crooked Councils, and dark Politicks. Pope

23. The Election Humbly Inscrib'd to the Saturday-Nights Club,
In Lodge Alley…Anonymous engraving, 1765.
A broadside, with a lengthy caption, reflecting opposition to
Benjamin Franklin's attitude toward the local government and the
loss of his seat in the Pennsylvania Assembly. There is nothing of
medical significance in the print itself, but one of the verses
discusses a quack doctor, and an advertisement proclaims the
efficacy of a "curry comb…if gently apply'd…will communicate
to the part Afflicted…" its magical properties. This product is
"To be sold…at the Bonnet and Broad Sword on So…ty Hill…
where Any Person, May be Supply'd with Rare Brimstone and
Butter, ready made up into Ointment, for the Same Begarly
Distemper." The verse pertaining to the quack doctor reads in part:

"The Blundering Doc..r, next doth mount the Stage
The Greatest Liar of The Present Age:
A Chymist Rare much Greater than a Boyle,
From Liv'r of Shark Draws twenty Quarts of Oil:
His Lies So oft Expos'd, to Publick View,
And told So often He Believ's them True:
Tis His to Weild, the Clyster Pipe and Launce,
To kill by Licence, or to Cure by Chance:"

Evans 9963; Murrell, I. p. 13

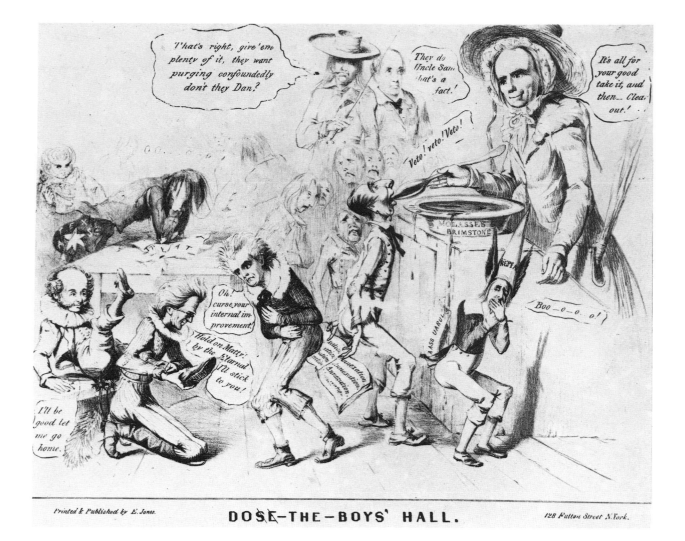

DOSE–THE–BOYS' HALL.

Printed & Published by E. Jones.   *128 Fulton Street N.York.*

24. Dose The Boys' Hall. Anonymous lithograph, 1844. One of the burning issues in the election of 1844 had to do with the annexation of Texas; this is one of the subjects treated in this anonymous lithograph. The subject is taken from Dickens' Nicholas Nickleby, and shows Clay administering

"Molasses and Brimstone" to Tyler. Among the other boys to be dosed are Van Buren and Jackson, one saying "Curse your internal improvement." Uncle Sam and Webster look on. agreeing that the boys "want purging confoundedly."

Weitenkampf, p. 81

drugs and pharmacy

Stimulants, purges and cathartics were the primary therapeutic agents used by physicians in the United States in the period up to 1870 and were frequently met with in the prints. They provided apt metaphors to the critics and cartoonists of the day for offering remedies to clean up the impurities of the political system. As early as 1765 an engraving commenting on local Philadelphia politics offered an ointment which was made up of "Rare Brimstone and Butter" (No. 23). It was Andrew Jackson's bank battle again, however, that provided the setting for several examples of this theme. Questions concerning the operations and influence of the Bank had been one of the major issues in the election of 1832. Before the election, Jackson and his supporters had opposed the conservative leadership of Nicholas Biddle, the Bank's president. They felt that the Bank has concentrated power in the hands of a few and had failed to establish a sound and uniform currency, and they championed a more liberal, "free money," policy. They supported measures designed to eliminate the Bank's charter and as a result,

by 1833, the case of the United States Bank was desperate indeed and the subject of much political turmoil. As one caricature, *The Doctors Puzzled or The Desperate Case of Mother U. S. Bank,* suggests, the Bank was a giant, or "monster," as it was called by its detractors (No. 5). Chief among these was the President himself and in the print he is seen peering in the window observing the discomfort of the Bank as well as of his political enemies. Jackson had vetoed the Congressional bill re-chartering the Bank and had ordered federal funds removed from it and placed in local banks. The effects of Jackson's "emetic" are clearly illustrated in the print as the Bank spews her vital coinage into basins labelled with the names of smaller, local banks. Straddling her shoulders is Nicholas Biddle, the Bank's president, enraged by the effects of Jackson's "prescription." John C. Calhoun, who recommends some "leaden pills of Nullification," and the other two attending physicians, Henry Clay and Daniel Webster are apparently unable to agree on how to counteract the violent regurgitation. At the time of the

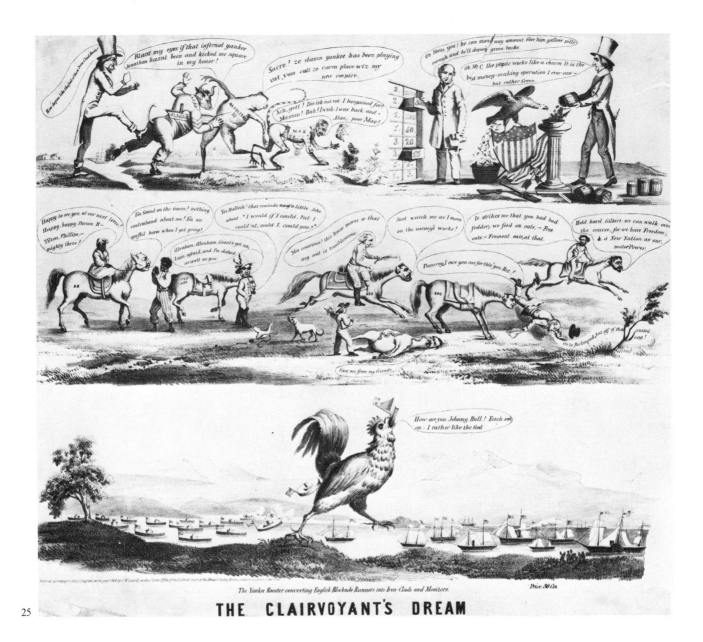

THE CLAIRVOYANT'S DREAM

25

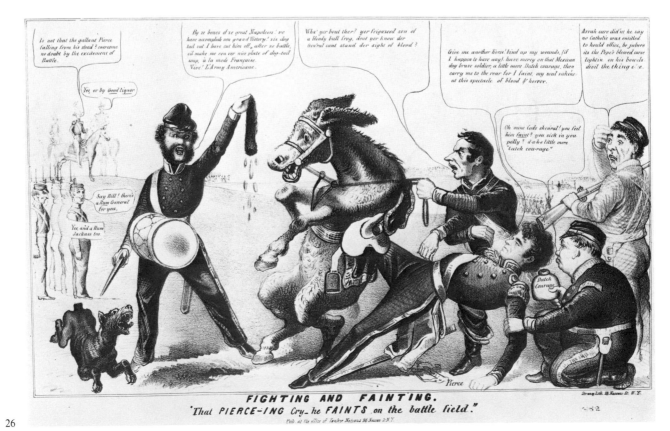

FIGHTING AND FAINTING.
"That PIERCE-ING Cry- he FAINTS on the battle field."

26

25. The Clairvoyant's Dream. Anonymous lithograph, 1864.
A print illustrating several ideas, one of which relates to the continuing economic difficulties in the North. In one part of this complicated print, Uncle Sam is shown feeding an eagle some "yellow pills." He tells Chase, (Salmon P. Chase, the Secretary of the Treasury) "Oh Mr. C. the physic works like a charm. It is the best money-making operation I ever saw—but rather Green." Chase comments "Oh Bless you! he can stand any amount. Give him yellow pills enough and he'll deposit green backs."

Weitenkampf, p. 147

26. Fighting and Fainting. Anonymous lithograph, 1852.
The election of 1852 was between Winfield Scott and Franklin Pierce. This print is a satire on Pierce, showing him falling from a horse on a battlefield. To revive him, an attendant offers a bottle of "Dutch Courage."

Weitenkampf, p. 111

27. Scene in the Tribune Office, New York.
Anonymous engraving, 1862.
Horace Greeley was one of the many thorns in Lincoln's side during the early months of the Civil War. In this print Greeley has fainted on news of a Union victory and has to be revived with some "Extract of Contracts."

From *Harper's Weekly*, Vol. 6, June 14, 1862, p. 384

28. The Great Union Prize Fight. Anonymous engraving, 1863.
A cartoon symbolizing the battle between the North and the South, showing Lincoln and Jefferson Davis engaged in a boxing match. As stimulants, attendants offer Lincoln a bottle labeled "The Arme of the Potomac," and Davis a bottle of "Braggs Victorie."

From New York Public Library

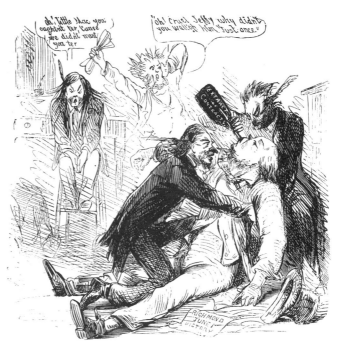

SCENE IN THE TRIBUNE OFFICE, NEW YORK.
Agony and Consternation caused by the receipt of News of another Victory by GENERAL McCLELLAN.

27

print these three were the major Whig opponents of Jackson and were in favor of the U. S. Bank's survival as a means of securing a stronger financial system for the country.

In other examples of the use of laxatives and cathartics to symbolize the elimination of problems at issue, Van Buren is given pills that are too purging, Henry Clay is shown administering molasses and brimstone and Uncle Sam is shown giving some physic in the form of yellow pills to an eagle (Nos. 13, 24, 25). Other agents used to accomplish this cleansing purpose for society in other prints were jalap, rhubarb, calomel, caster oil and croton oil. But laxatives were not the only type of pharmaceutical product to be employed as a therapeutic measure. Stimulants were offered for the fainting spells suffered by Franklin Pierce (No. 26) and Horace Greeley (No. 27), and they were also employed in one print illustrating a boxing match be-

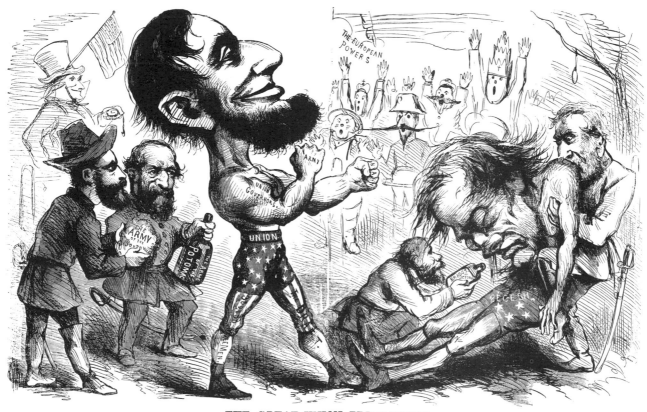

THE GREAT UNION PRIZE FIGHT.

JEFF. DAVIS.---I've whipped you in every round, and now I think you'd bett.t give up, and come to my terms.
LINCOLN, comes up smiling---No, no; I'll fight it out. I never felt stronger than I do now. Come on, and I'll give you a finishing touch.
UNCLE SAM, referee---Your time is nearly up.

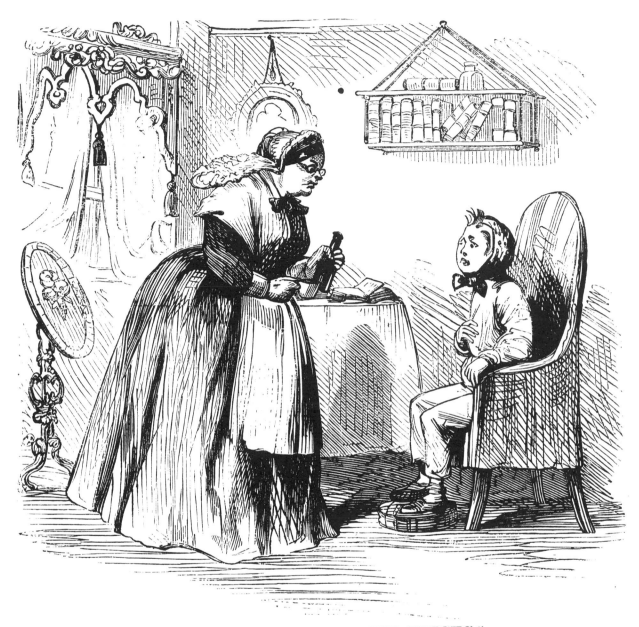

ADVANTAGE OF "FAMINE PRICES."

SICK BOY. "I know one thing—I wish I was in Dixie."

NURSE. "And why do you wish you was in Dixie, you wicked boy?"

SICK BOY. "Because I read that quinine is worth one hundred and fifty dollars an ounce there; and if it was that here you wouldn't pitch it into me so!"

29. Advantage of "Famine Prices." Anonymous engraving, 1863.
A comment on economic problems. The print shows a nurse giving
a sick boy some quinine.

From *Harper's Weekly*, Vol. 7, Nov. 4, 1863, p. 736

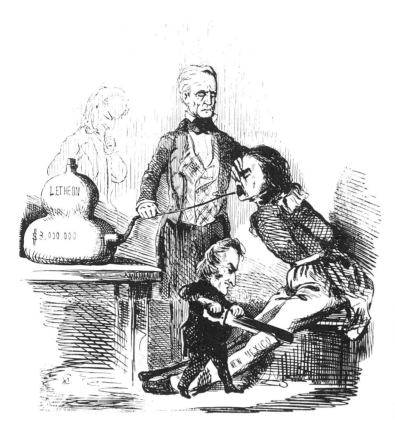

TRIUMPH OF THE LETHEON.

30. Triumph of the Letheon. Anonymous engraving, 1847.
A print on the Mexican War in Polk's administration. An amputation is being performed while the patient is inhaling an anesthetic. The text to the print notes, "Doctor Tom Thumb Benton reports a remarkable case, in which he removed a leg from a distinguished Mexican General while under the influence of a new variety of the Letheon discovered by a well-known political-chemist, Mr. Polk. This form of the Letheon is very expensive, the present dose having cost $3,000,000. Dr. Benton says that the General is even now unconscious of having lost his other leg . . . . it is said that Mr. Polk after copious inhalations is able to think upon the Mexican War with feelings approaching to complacency."

From *Yankee Doodle*, Vol. 2, 1847, p. 5

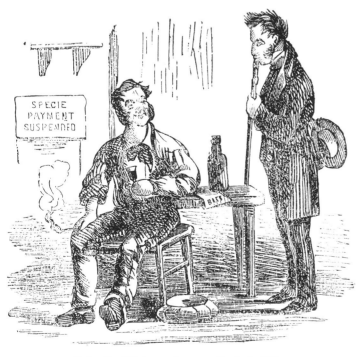

Take the Hint ye who owe Doctor's Bills.

Patient.—AH, AS TO YOUR LITTLE ITEMS, TO VISITS AND MIXTURES, DOCTOR, I'LL RETURN YOUR VISITS, AND IF YE'LL HONOR ME WID YER COMPANY AT DINNER TO-MORROW, I'LL GIVE YOU MORE PALATABLE MIXTURES THAN THOSE I RECEIVED.

31. Take the Hint ye who owe Doctor's Bills.
Anonymous engraving, 1858.
A comment on the financial problems of the country in Buchanan's term in office. The print shows a seated patient talking to a physician. The caption indicates that the patient will return the doctor's visits and "give you more palatable mixtures than those I received." On the table is the doctor's "Bill."

From *Yankee Notions*, Vol. 7, Feb., 1858, p. 45

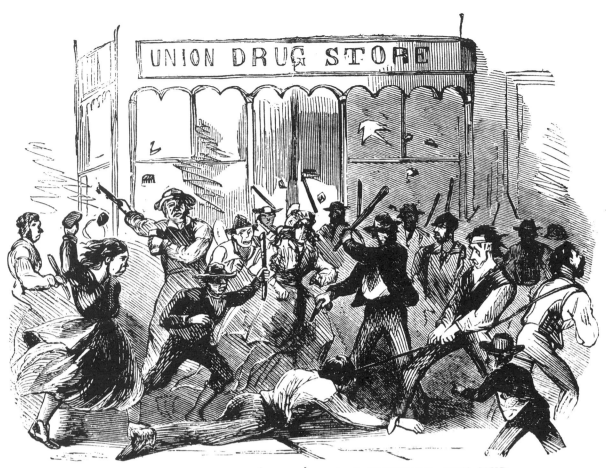

DRAGGING COLONEL O'BRIEN'S BODY THROUGH THE MUD.

32

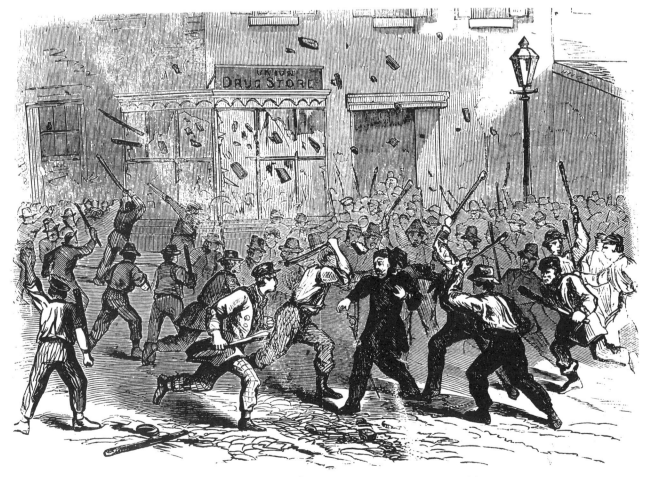

BRUTAL MURDER OF COL. H. F. O'BRIEN, NEAR HIS REST   JULY 14.

33

tween Lincoln and Jefferson Davis (No. 28), representing the two sides in the War Between the States. Quinine figures in one Civil War print (No. 29), and iron, the symbol of fortitude, is recommended in two others (Nos. 20 and 2). Anesthesia was the subject of a print published in 1847, the *Triumph of the Letheon*, a timely reference to Morton's proposed patent of the previous year[5] (No. 30). The bad taste of medicines is alluded to in one print (No. 31), this being a theme which had its counterparts in prints published in Europe during the eighteenth and nineteenth centuries.

The drug store was the setting for a number of political comments during the period covered, mainly after 1860. The exterior of a drug store is noticeable in several prints, three of which show a pharmacy as incidental background to illustrations of the draft riots in New York in 1863 (Nos. 32, 33, 34). In general, the pharmacy provided the caricaturist with a convenient place to present a case for his own political nostrum. To make his point, the artist often drew satirically, with tongue in cheek, in his efforts to illustrate his own point of view. One example of these prints using the pharmacy as a setting, Delusive Druggist, concerns Lincoln's beard (No. 35). In the politics of 1861, personal appearance and mannerisms were as subject to editorial comment as they have always been and still are today. A pharmacist urges a clean-shaven customer to purchase some sort of medication which will enable him to grow a beard like Lincoln's. The pharmacist promises that in three weeks the young man will be as "'airy and 'ansom as 'im," pointing to Lincoln. Soon after the election of 1860 Lincoln grew a beard but his political adversaries were not deterred by the facial camouflage. During his political career Loncoln was ridiculed for his homely features and gangly stature in much the same way that President Gerald Ford had been chided for his alleged clumsiness.

5. Fielding H. Garrison. *An Introduction to the History of Medicine*, W. B. Saunders Co., Philadelphia, 1924. ed. 3, p. 541

32. Dragging Colonel O'Brien's Body Through the Mud.
Anonymous engraving, 1863.
A print to illustrate an article on the draft riots in New York in 1863. The print shows rioters in front of a drug store.

From *Harper's Weekly*, Vol. 7, Aug. 1, 1863, p. 485

33. Brutal Murder of Col. H. F. O'Brien, Near his Residence.
Anonymous engraving, 1863.
The same subject as the previous print, showing the fighting taking place in front of a drug store.

From *Frank Leslie's Illustrated Newspaper*, Vol. 16, Aug. 1, 1863. p. 300

34. Sacking a Drug Store in Second Avenue.
Anonymous engraving, 1863.
Another print on the draft riots, showing the rioters looting a pharmacy.

From *Harper's Weekly*, Vol. 7, Aug. 1, 1863, p. 484

SACKING A DRUG STORE IN SECOND AVENUE.

34

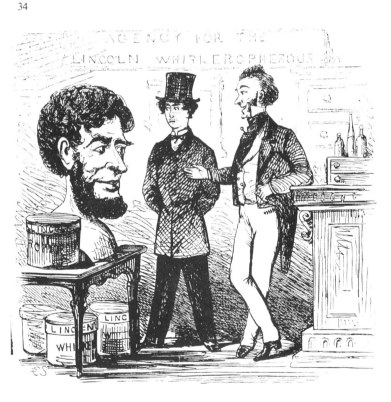

Delusive Druggist.—THERE'S 'IS EFFIGY IN WAX, SIR, WISKERS AND ALL. TRY ONE OF THEM POTS, AND IN THREE WEEKS YOU'LL BE AS 'AIRY AND 'ANSOM AS 'IM.

35. Delusive Druggist. Anonymous engraving, 1861.
A cartoon commenting on Lincoln's new beard, grown only after the election was over. In a pharmacy is a bust of a bearded Lincoln; a sign on the wall notes that it is an "Agency for the Lincoln Whiskeropherous." The druggist leans on a counter on which are some bottles of medicine.

From *Vanity Fair*, Vol. 3, Mar. 16, 1861, p. 126; Shaw, p. 109; Wilson, p. 113

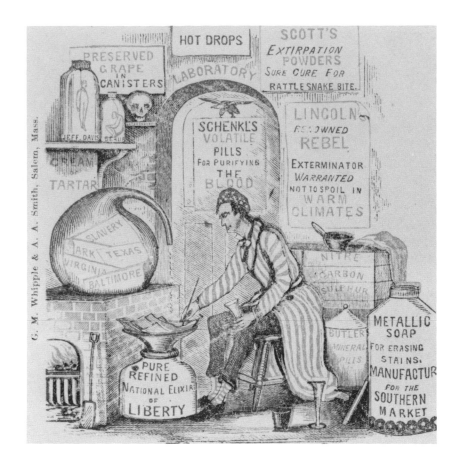

36. Lincoln's Laboratory. A series of advertising signs for various drug products surround Lincoln as he is shown manufacturing some "Elixir of Liberty."

From W. H. Helfand Collection

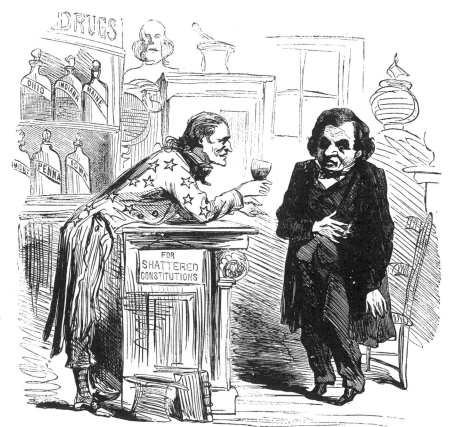

Extract Const. Amend.

"Now, ANDY, take it right down. More you Look at it, worse you'll Like it."

37. Extract Const. Amend. Anonymous engraving, 1866.
Johnson's difficulties are the subject of this cartoon, which shows Uncle Sam as a pharmacist, behind the counter of his drug store. He offers some medicine to Andrew Johnson, along with some advice. A sign on the counter notes that the medicine is "For Shattered Constitutions."

From *Harper's Weekly*, Vol. 10, Oct. 27, 1866, p. 688

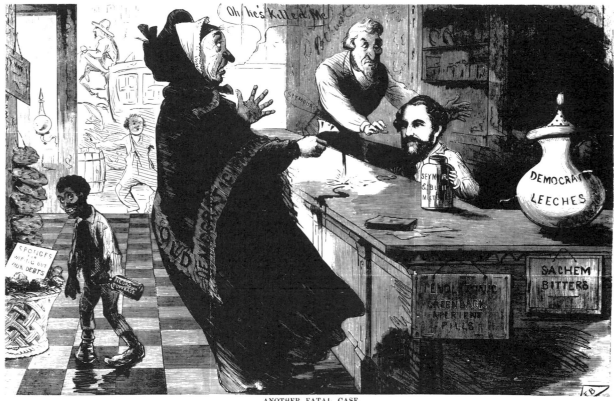

ANOTHER FATAL CASE.

OLD APOTHECARY—", YE YOUNG FULF, PENDLETON, YE'VE JUST POISONED THE PUIR AULD BODY! SHE'LL NEVER GET OVER THAT DOSE."

38. Another Fatal Case. Engraving by Frank Bellew, 1868.
A pro-Republican 1868 election print. Behind the counter of a
drug store are Seymour, the candidate, and James Gordon
Bennett, the editor. A woman, depicting the "Old Democratic
Party," has taken a drink from a cup of "Seymour's Drops," and
been poisoned. A boy holds a bottle of medicine labeled "Negro
Suffrage"; other signs advertise "Pendletonic Greenback
Aperient Pills," and "Sachem Bitters." On the counter
is a jar of "Democratic Leeches" and a bottle of "Seymour &
Blair Mixture."

From Historical Society of Pennsylvania

In other prints, Lincoln himself is the pharmacist
(No. 36), and this professional role was also played by
Uncle Sam, James Gordon Bennett, and Horatio Seymour, Grant's rival in the presidential campaign of
1868 (Nos. 37 and 38). In the print, *A Bitter "Draught"*
a small card printed in 1863, Lincoln is shown offering
this remedy from a bowl labeled "Conscription" (No.
39). A sign on a wall of his pharmacy advertising "Dr.
Lincoln's Ready Relief Pills," shows examples of the
product itself. When the print was issued, the Civil
War was raging and military conscription was provid-
ing manpower for the war effort. The poor were most
susceptible to the draft because they were unable to
purchase deferments as could many well-to-do men, a
situation referred to in other prints and caricatures of
the period. In the northern cities of nineteenth century
America, to be Irish generally was to be poor. Politically, the Irish were Democrats, and they bitterly re-

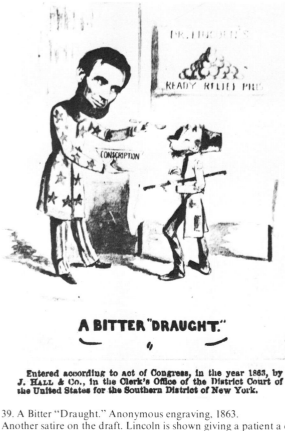

A BITTER "DRAUGHT."

Entered according to Act of Congress, in the year 1863, by
J. HALL & Co., in the Clerk's Office of the District Court of
the United States for the Southern District of New York.

39. A Bitter "Draught." Anonymous engraving, 1863.
Another satire on the draft. Lincoln is shown giving a patient a dose
from a bottle labeled "Conscription." A sign on a wall advertised
"Dr. Lincoln's Ready Relief Pills."

From Historical Society of Pennsylvania

31

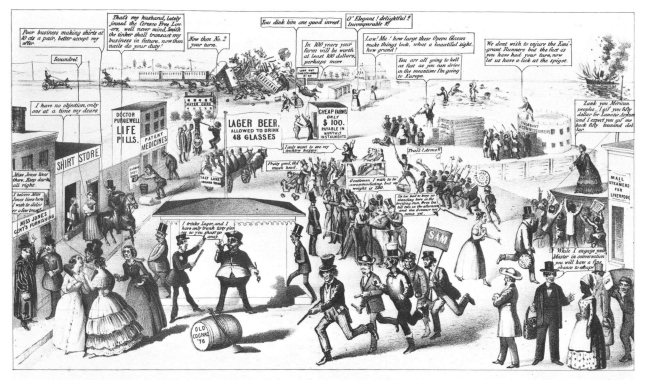

THE FOLLIES OF THE AGE, VIVE LA HUMBUG!!

40. The Follies of the Age, Vive la Humbug!! Anonymous lithograph, c. 1852.
Comments on a series of aspects of life in the United States in the 1850's are
presented in this conglomerate print. Included are satires on Mormons,
remedies, women, etc. One of the buildings shown carries signs for "Patent
Medicines" and "Doctor Purgewell Life Pills." Another building nearby
advertises "Water Cure."

Weitenkampf, p. 100

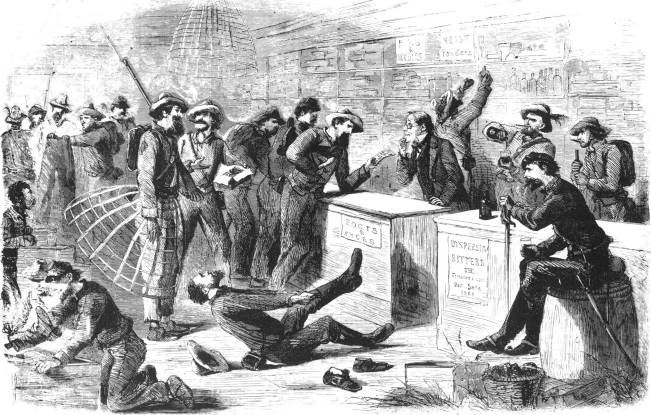

REBELS SHOPPING IN PENNSYLVANIA.

41. Rebels Shopping in Pennsylvania. Anonymous engraving, 1863.
This print illustrates a group of soldiers in a general store. There are signs in
the store advertising "Yeast Powders" and "Dyspepsia Bitters."

New York Illustrated News, vol. 8, July 18, 1863, p. 185.

sented the draft, declaring they were being forced to fight a war of Republican making. As a result, the widespread rioting in Northern cities was heavily Irish. The stereotypical caricature of the shillelagh-toting Irishman being spooned the bitter draught of conscription by "Dr." Lincoln in the cartoon well illustrates the caricaturist's view of the system.

Several of the prints show the mortar and pestle, and many of them have, usually as part of the background, some advertisements for patent medicines or quack nostrums. These cover a wide range, and include, among others, "Dr. Purgewell Life Pills" (No. 40) "Dr. Hickory's Celebrated Cure for Corns" (No. 22) "Yeast Powders" (No. 41) "Dyspepsia Bitters" (No. 41) "Sachem Bitters" (No. 38) and "Pendleton's Greenback Aperient Pills" (No. 38). In addition to "Dr. Lincoln's Ready Relief Pills," already referred to there are two other nostrums offered by Lincoln, his "Whiskeropherous" (No. 35), and his "Specific for Confederate Rash" (No. 42). One 1861 lithograph contains signs for three nostrums, "Bond Plasters," "Great Southern Remedies" and "Dr. Jeffy's Celebrated Lettres du Marque," a product that is advertised to stimulate the blood, excite action and elevate the patient (No. 43).

Throughout these prints other medicines, some authentic, but most completely fictional in nature, are employed to produce some political result. The legitimate drugs are few, and include the iron, jalap, quinine, castor oil and rhubarb already noted. But the imaginary medicines are more varied and creative as the following list would indicate, the bitters appear in several forms, as Cholera, Secession and Lowell; there are Black, and Last Southern Draughts; there are Mint, Constitution, Benton and Seymour's Drops. The list of pills is even broader, including Blue, Yellow, Dinner, Gold, Leaden, Pickpock and Poinsett's Indian. Liquid medications include Winslow, Greely's, and just plain Soothing Syrups, Weed's Elixir, the Elixir of Life, Milk Sop, Sub-Treasury Pap, African Pap, Pennsylvania Gruel and Seward's Gruel. The list goes on— Calhoun's Loco Foco Life Preserver, Poke-berry Juice, Juice of Humbug, Bank Cordial, Dysentery Cordial, Russian Salve, Dr. Dugan's Soporific, Spirit of Cave-In, etc. The imagination of the coiners of these and other political trademarks was broad indeed, for in the majority of cases, these panaceas were designed to provide relief or cure for the burning political problems of the moment.

42. Drawing Things to a Head. Anonymous engraving, 1863.
By the time of this cartoon, the Union forces had begun to take command, and their victory looked certain. The print shows Lincoln as a doctor in a pharmacy telling his errand boy, Secretary of State Wm. H. Seward, who carries a basket containing some "Russia Salve," his prescription. A sign in the shop advertises "Dr. Lincoln's specific for Confederate Rash [-] Russia Salve," and another identifies "Ericsson Monitor Galvanic Battery." There is also a large clyster labeled "Parrot's Syringe."

From *Harper's Weekly*, Vol. 7, Nov. 28, 1863, p. 768; Wilson, p. 257

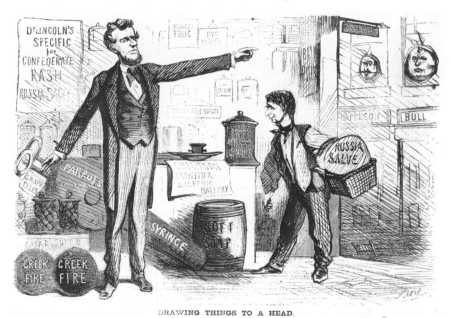

DRAWING THINGS TO A HEAD.

Dr. Lincoln (*to Smart Boy of the Shop*). "Mild applications of Russian Salve for our *friends* over the way, and heavy doses—and plenty of it—for our Southern patient!!"

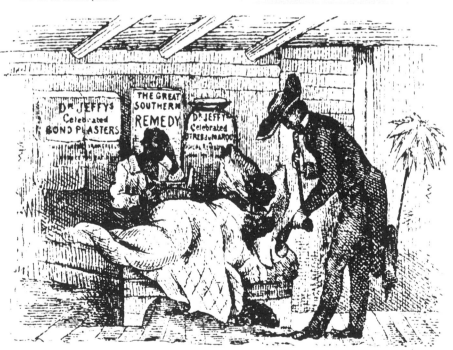

Oh! Massa Jeff. dis Sesesh Fever will kill de Nigger

43. Oh! Massa Jeff. dis Sesesh Fever will kill de Nigger.
Anonymous lithograph, 1861.
This caricature is one of the many designed as satire against the South. It shows Jefferson Davis, as a doctor, feeling the pulse of a negro in bed with the words "Bond Plasters" on his chest. Another negro in attendance holds a bottle of medicine. On the wall are three signs, for "Bond Plasters," "The Great Southern Remedies," and "Dr. Jeffy's Celebrated Lettres du Marque, A Radical Remedy for all Constitutional Affections. It Stimulates the Blood, Excites Action and Elevates the Patient...." This print also appeared on one of the Civil War Envelopes (see No. 54).

Weitenkampf, p. 128

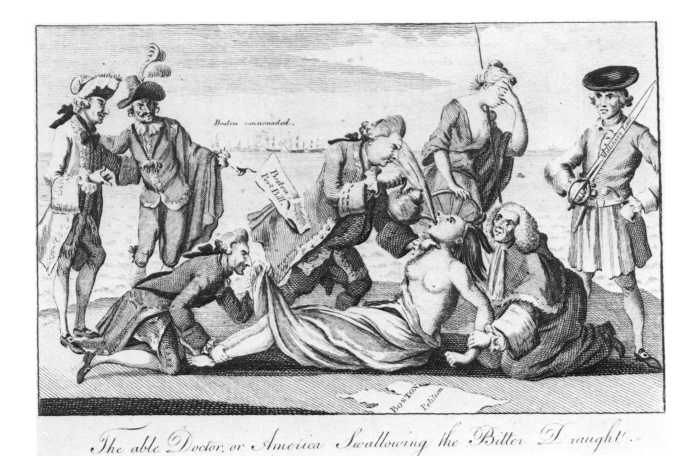

Boston cannonaded.

Boston Port Bill.

BOSTON Petition.

The able Doctor, or America Swallowing the Bitter Draught.

44. The able Doctor, or America Swallowing the Bitter Draught. Engraving by Paul Revere, 1774.
A print from the *Royal American Magazine,* June, 1774, copied from the *London Magazine,* April, 1774, and commenting on the Boston Port Bill. The original British print shows Bute, North and other British statesmen forcing a woman representing America to

drink the bitter medicine while the Kings of France and Spain watch. Revere has altered the print only to have the medicine come from a pitcher of "tea."

Brigham, pp. 85-87; George (1959), I , p. 150; Hess & Kaplan, p. 187; Tyler, p. 47

administration of medicine

Perhaps the most frequent medical image of all showed a physician (or a nurse), in the act of giving medicine to a sick patient, or the patients taking medicines themselves without benefit of professional aid. Two early Paul Revere engravings, copies of prints that had appeared earlier in London, for example, show a group of physicians administering to the ills of America by pouring their remedy, tea, down the throat of the patient (Nos. 44 and 45). One of the prints published as propaganda for the North in 1861, *Oh! Massa Jeff…* has slavery itself as the ailing subject (No. 43). There were many who, even in the face of Southern secession, called slavery a dying institution. Slavery they contended, if allowed to run its natural course in the South, would die quietly of economic causes, its days were numbered. Thus in the print, Jefferson Davis, President of the Confederate States of America, is shown taking the pulse of a desperately ill slave. His remedies include "Bond Plasters"—war bonds—and "Lettres du Marque"—commissions given to private ships to act as Confederate gunboats. But Davis' cure for the "ailing" patient does not seem to be working in the eyes of the cartoonist.

Other "doctors" involved in the therapeutic act during the period up to 1870 included Lincoln, Grant, Johnson, and the U.S. Congress itself. There were also cartoons commenting on the European scene. For example, a copy of an engraving by the British caricaturist, John Leech, appeared in *Harper's Weekly* showing France, (symbolized by the Emperor Napoleon III) as the doctor along with a shelf full of medicine bottles that had been prescribed for the Pope and Sultan of Turkey (No. 46). Besides physicians, nurses also were shown administering medicines. In *The Constitution and its Nurses,* for example, there are seven Democratic leaders attending the patient, and the print affords some insight into the politics of the 1840's (No. 47). Western expansion, the swelling population of the Eastern States, and the upsurge of American industry and commerce brought about fierce political rivalries. Factions of varied interests were clamoring for control.

In the midst of all that was changing, the Constitution represented the unalterable ideals of the American polity and no administration would move without some sort of statement proclaiming the constitutionality of its intended actions. Of course, the matter of

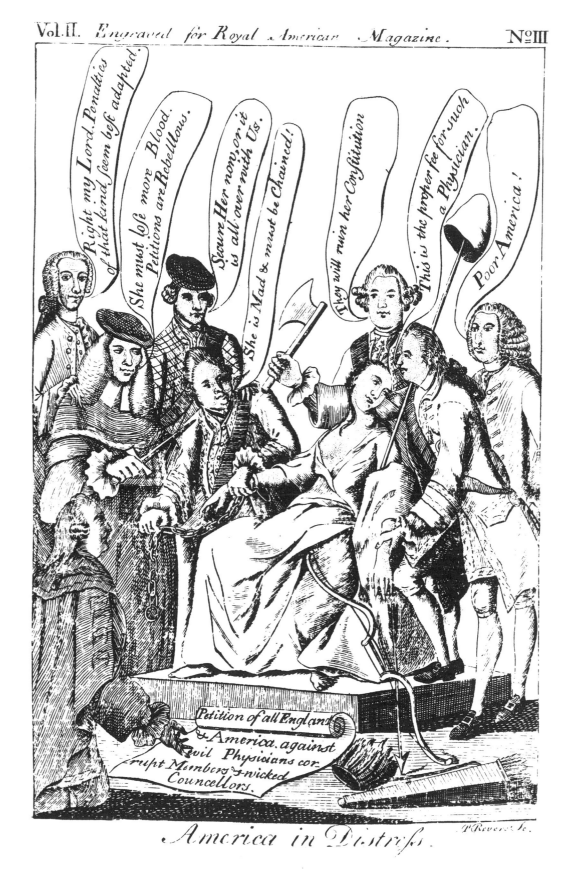

45. America in Distress. Engraving by Paul Revere, 1775.
A print from the *Royal American Magazine*, March, 1775, copied from the *Oxford Magazine*, February, 1770. Although the original print commented on several contemporary British problems, Revere altered it slightly, in both the figures presented and the captions used, to depict some of the evils besetting the colonies just prior to the War for Independence. America is shown surrounded by a group of physicians who are both diagnosing her ills and prescribing their suggested treatments.

Brigham, pp. 90-91; Stevens and Hawkins, p. 602

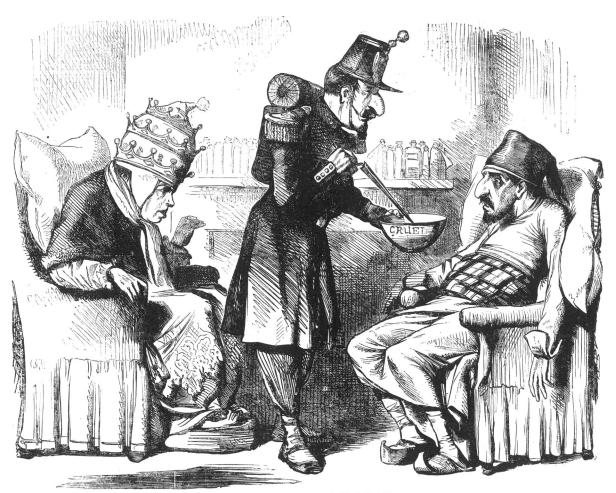

THE TWO SICK MEN.

POPE.——"They have sent you my French Doctor, I see. His Course of Steel hasn't done *my* System much Good."

THE TWO SICK MEN.

In Europe two sick men do dwell,
Of whom there's little hope;
The SULTAN one: as far from well
The other is the POPE.
This wreck a triple crown, and that
A Royal turban wears;
Too weak the head in either hat
To manage its affairs.

The first has been a sufferer sad
For many a weary day;

And loads of physic he has had
To keep grim Death at bay.
The second 'gan to limp and reel
Some dozen years ago,
When his French doctor threw in steel;
Maintained his system so.

Eruptions, here and there, about
Each leper's surface rage;
And either is well nigh worn out
By frequent hæmorrhage.

Yet their physician still declares
That both must more be bled,
And take more steel, by which he swears,
Exhibited with lead.

The POPE cries, "Heathen friend, I see
You've got my doctor too;
He hasn't done much good to me,
May he do more to you!"
"My Giaour," the groaning TURK replies,
"We're past physician's skill;

To cure us if your doctor tries
He'll all the sooner kill."

Gone are both systems to decay,
Effete old POPE and TURK!
No Constitution left have they
Whereon the Leech might work.
Could they but break up quietly,
And leave the world in peace,
Blest would the dissolution be,
And happy the release.

46

46. The Two Sick Men.
Engraving by John Leech, 1860.
European problems are the subject of this print, which was taken from a cartoon in *Punch*, the British humor magazine. It shows France, as a physician, administering "Gruel" to the Pope and the Sultan of Turkey. A long row of medicine bottles is on a mantelpiece.

From *Harper's Weekly*, Vol. 4, Sept. 15, 1860, p. 592

47. The Constitution and its Nurses.
Anonymous lithograph, c. 1847.
Comments on political activity of the Democrats at the time of the campaign between Cass and Tyler are shown in this print. Here, Van Buren, Jackson, Polk, Tyler, Clay, Cass and Johnson, are all depicted as nurses ministering to the nation. Polk holds a bottle of "Anti-Tarif"; Clay also holds a bottle to give to the baby.

From American Antiquarian Society

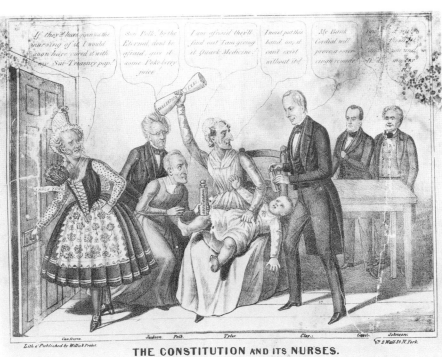

47

THE CONSTITUTION AND ITS NURSES.

"constitutionality" was open to interpretation and amendment. Thus, in the print of *The Constitution and its Nurses* (No. 47) the Constitution is portrayed as a helpless baby being ministered to by four Presidents and a Senator. Holding the baby is John Tyler, President from 1841-1845. He was instrumental in annexing the State of Texas, an act his own party was firmly against. On his right is James Polk, President from 1845-1849. Polk, a political scion of "Old Hickory," who stands closely behind him, tries to feed the Constitution an "Anti-Tarif" bill. The tariff was unpopular among Southern merchants and so became an important target for Southern Democrats like Jackson and Polk. Van Buren, another President (1837-1841), is seen leaving the room, probably in reference to his own party's rejection of him as its candidate in 1840. He wants to nurse the Constitution with an amendment to establish an independent Federal treasury. Standing to the right of Tyler is Henry Clay, the Senator from Kentucky, who although a Presidential hopeful for many years, never attained the office. The bottle he wishes to feed the Constitution is a bill to reestablish the Bank of the United States, something he also failed to achieve. Lewis Cass, the Democratic nominee for the 1848 presidential election, stands in the background, eagerly awaiting his chance to "feed the baby" his own formula.

foreign influences

As the list of prints relevant to our subject indicates, there are 37 examples that were issued prior to 1860, and more than 70 that appeared during the 1860's, excluding those designed for use as propaganda on envelopes during the Civil War (See p. 82 and Nos. 48-60 and 36).[6] The existence of this group of pre-1860 political caricatures using medicine and pharmacy as background points up an exception to Leake's contention that "The gentle art of caricature did not develop in the United States until the Civil War period,"[7] and that "The first strictly medical caricature published in this country came out in Harper's Weekly in 1858."[8]

However, the number of political prints of medical interest issued in the United States was far less than the production in England and France during the same interval. In the period to 1835, not includ-

6. William H. Helfand, "Pharmaceutical Themes on Patriotic Envelopes."
   Journal of the American Pharmaceutical Assn.,
   1970, NS 10, 7, 418
7. Chauncey D. Leake, "Medical Caricature in the United States."
   Bull. Soc. Med. Hist. Chicago, 1928, IV, 1.3
8. *Ibid,* p.9

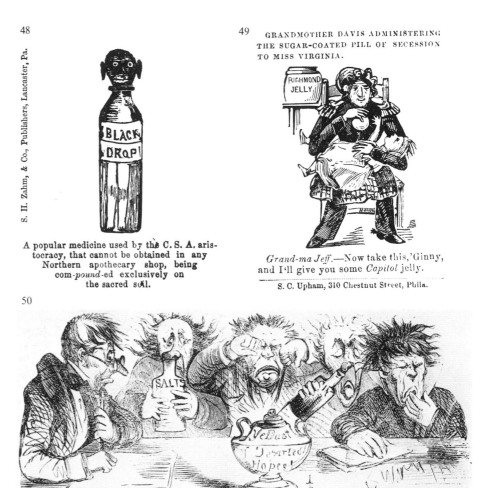

48

S. H. Zahm, & Co., Publishers, Lancaster, Pa.

A popular medicine used by the C. S. A. aristocracy, that cannot be obtained in any Northern apothecary shop, being com-*pound*-ed exclusively on the sacred s❍il.

49 GRANDMOTHER DAVIS ADMINISTERING THE SUGAR-COATED PILL OF SECESSION TO MISS VIRGINIA.

Grand-ma Jeff.—Now take this, 'Ginny, and I'll give you some *Capitol* jelly.

S. C. Upham, 310 Chestnut Street, Phila.

50

A CONVENTION OF SECESSIONISTS AFTER THE WAR.

51

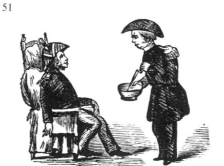

J. D. (patient.) Doctor, I don't know what to think of my disorder. I should call it the *ague*, only the fever came *first*, and now I am shaking in my boots.
Dr. Scott. Well, Davis, you'll find you are too far north. You will have the *shakes* in earnest unless you take some of this *Union Broth* to strengthen you—you must take it!

S. C. Upham, 310 Chestnut St.

52 THE FOX AND THE GOOSE.

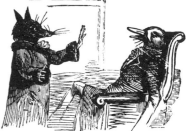

Wm. Redenburgh, 140 Nassau Street, N. Y.

Well, my dear Governor, how do you feel now? Ah! Dr. Davis, that last secession pill will be the death of me—and Old Virginia too, I fear

48. Black Drop. A bottle of medicine with a black man as the cork.

Helfand, p. 419

49. Grandmother Davis Administering the Sugar-Coated Pill of Secession to Miss Virginia. Davis is shown giving a huge bolus to a little girl; a jar of "Richmond Jelly" is in the background, offered as a reward for the girl's taking the pill.

Helfand, p. 418

50. A Convention of Secessionists After the War. A group of five men at a table, two of whom require the use of "salts."

Helfand, p. 419

51. "Doctor, I don't know what to think of my disorder...." General Winfield Scott, as a physician, recommends some "Union Broth" to his patient, Jefferson Davis.

Helfand, p. 419

52. The Fox and the Goose. Here Jefferson Davis, as a fox, is the physician, and the patient states that secession will be the death of "me—and old Virginia too...."

Helfand, p. 418

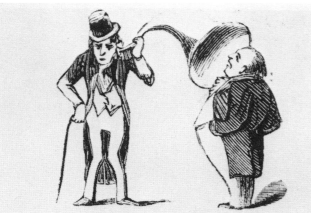

Deaf Man—I have got the Secession Fever, and it is making me deaf.
Union Man—Get some of Magee's Union Envelopes, and that will cure you of the fever.

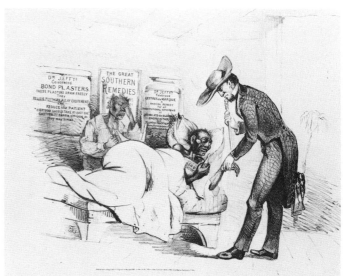

Oh! Massa Jeff. dis Sesesh Fever will kill de Nigger

53. "I have got the Secession Fever, and it is making me deaf."
A deaf man, with a huge ear trumpet is addressed by a "Union Man" who recommends a cure.

Hess & Kaplan, p. 29; Helfand, p. 419

54. Oh! Massa Jeff, dis Sesesh Fever will kill de Nigger. A small reproduction of a cartoon that was published separately (see No. 43).

From W. H. Helfand Collection.

55. One of the F.F.V.'s, Colonel of the Dysentery Blue….The F.F.V.'s referred to the First Families of Virginia, and the illustration of a Confederate general is a reference to the unfortunate General Stirling Price (see Nos. 87, 88 and 92).

From W. H. Helfand Collection

56. Secession Physic Cure. An illustration of a bottle of "Union Bitters," "Dr. Scott's Pills," and a "powder" with a six-line verse recommending these ingredients "To cure Secession and its ills."

Dannett, p. 127; Helfand, p. 419

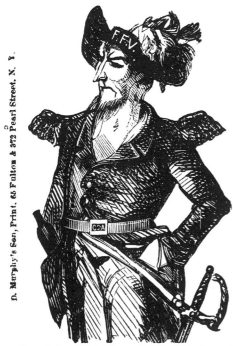

One of the F. F. V's, Colonel of the Dysentery Blues who thinks his martial appearance will strike terror into the hearts of the "Northern mudsills."

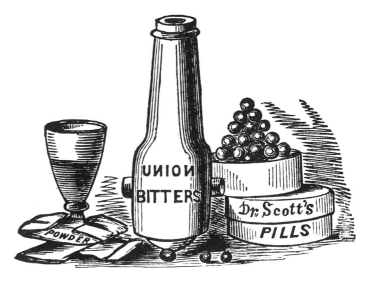

SECESSION PHYSIC CURE.

To cure *Secession* and its ills,
Take Dr. Scott's *Cast Iron Pills*;
Well mixed with *Powder* of *Saltpetre*,
Apply it to each "*Fire Eater*."
With *Union Bitters*, mix it clever,
And *treason* is warned off forever.

TO CURE REBELLION.

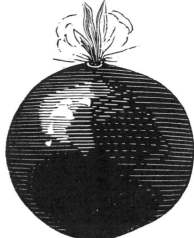

'This is the Pill that will Cure or Kill.'

57. To Cure Rebellion. A bomb is recommended as "…the Pill that will Cure or Kill."

From W. H. Helfand Collection

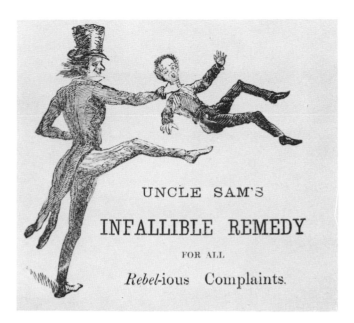

UNCLE SAM'S

INFALLIBLE REMEDY

FOR ALL

Rebel-ious Complaints.

58. Uncle Sam's Infallible Remedy for all *Rebel*-ious Complaints. The illustration shows Uncle Sam kicking a rather small complainer.

Helfand, p. 418

59. Uncle Sam's Recipe for Traitors. Uncle Sam holds a bottle marked "Davis," with the directions advising that it is "To be Well Shaken Before Taken."

Helfand, p. 418

60. The "Union" Pill in operation, working out the quack nostrums of Doctor Davis & Co. The cartoon shows a fight between a large pill marked "Union" with some rival panaceas labeled "Confederated Mixture," "Secession Pills" and "Davis Lotion."

Helfand, p. 419

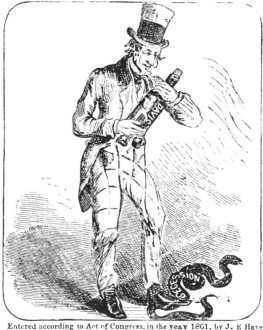

Entered according to Act of Congress, in the year 1861, by J. E Hayes in the Clerk's Office in the District Court of the District of Massachusetts.

Uncle Sam's Recipe for Traitors.

"TO BE WELL SHAKEN BEFORE TAKEN."

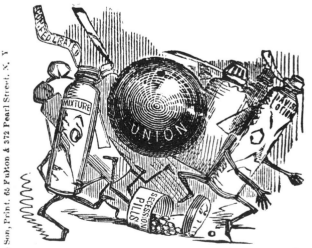

D. Murphy & Son, Print. 65 Fulton & 372 Pearl Street, N. Y.

The "Union" Pill in operation, working out the quack nostrums of Doctor Davis & Co.

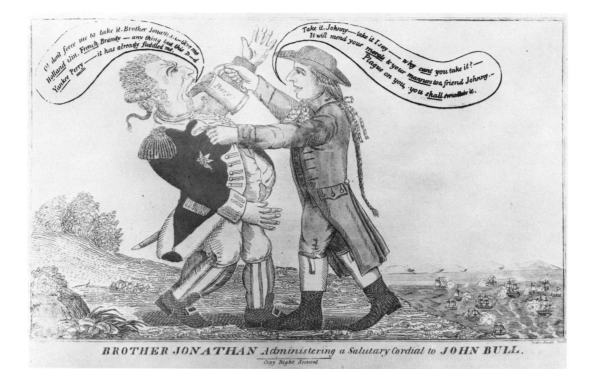

61. Brother Jonathan Administering a Salutary Cordial to John Bull.
Engraving by Amos Doolittle, 1813.
A print discussing the triumphs of Captain Oliver H. Perry over British ships
in the Battle of Lake Erie. Brother Jonathan, representing the United States,
is shown pouring the contents of a mug labeled "Perry" down the throat of
John Bull.

Murrell I, pp. 60-62; Weitenkampf, p. 17; Dreppard, p. 212; Hess and
Kaplan, p. 34; Foreign Policy Assn., p. 9

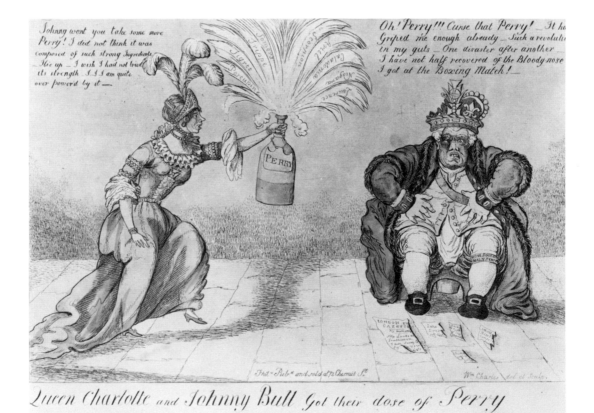

62. Queen Charlotte and Johnny Bull Got Their Dose of Perry.
Engraving by William Charles, 1813.
This engraving treats the same subject as No. 61 by showing the Queen
handling a bottle of "Perry" to the King, shown seated on a commode.

Weitenkampf, p. 17; Dreppard, p. 212; Murrell, I, pp. 88-89; Hess & Kaplan,
p. 64; Foreign Policy Assn., p. 10

ing the examples in serial publications during the next 35 years, over 400 British political caricatures dealing with medicine and pharmacy have been catalogued. Daumier alone, as an example of French production, used these professions as background for more than 50 lithographs relating to political subjects. The art of caricature, at least up to 1870, in other countries including Germany, Russia and Spain, was about as developed as our own; none of these could rival England and France in either quantity or quality of effort. Because the political cartoonist is most concerned about domestic matters of immediate impact, it is not surprising that very little of this large British and French output pertains to America, but the few exceptions are not too different in approach from our own domestic offerings.

An example of an eighteenth century French print with some American interest is *L'anglois a Toute Extremité*, a 1778 engraving illustrating America's victories over England. In political subject, it is quite similar to Nos. 61 and 62; and in medical subject, that of an apothecary (Benjamin Franklin) administering a clyster to a patient (England), it is close to the subject of No. 8. Another British print of 1782 refers to peace with America and shows one member of the ministry, Lord Rockingham, as an oculist.[9] Two British cartoons issued at the time of the Civil War also paralleled American examples, John Tenniel's *The Black Draft*[10] shows two soldiers given medicine by orderlies, Lincoln and Jefferson Davis, a subject close to that of Nos. 63 and 39. And Matt Morgan's *After His Last Run,*[11] showing Lincoln as a physician administering to General McClellan, a patient with his feet in a bucket of hot water, is remarkably similar to the American examples as shown in Nos. 11 and 12.

Also, with the extensive British and later the French experience to guide them, much of the American output is reminiscent of earlier foreign effort in the period covered. Paul Revere's copying of two British engravings (Nos. 44 and 45) is perhaps the most direct example of this influence, but William Charles' engraving of *Queen Charlotte and Johnny Bull Get Their Dose of Perry* (No. 62) is quite close to the efforts of James Gillray, an artist whose works Charles imitates closely.[12] William Charles had issued a number of caricatures in England prior to his emigration to the United States. Finally, many of the works of Henry L. Stephens, William Newman and Frank Bellew of the Civil War period are similar in nature to the efforts of John Leech, John Tenniel and Matt Morgan which had appeared in earlier issues of the British humor weeklies, *Punch* and *Fun*.

9. Mary Dorothy George, "America in English Satirical Prints,"
   Wm. & Mary Q., 1953, 3rd Ser., X, (4), p. 530
10. *Punch,* Nov. 19, 1864
11. *Fun,* Aug. 2, 1862
12. Stephen Hess and Milton Kaplan, *The Ungentlemanly Art,*
   The MacMillan Co., New York, 1968, p. 62

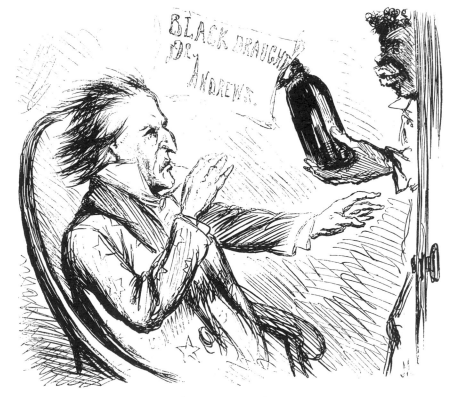

BLACK DRAFT.

Colored Person.—" DOCTOR ANDREW'S COMPLUMS, MASSA; AND HE SAYS YOU MUST SWALLER DIS HERE STUFF."

Uncle Sam.—" UGH ! TAKE THE NASTY THING AWAY ! I'M SICK ENOUGH ALREADY !"

63. Black Draft. Anonymous engraving, 1862.
The draft of soldiers and the draught as medicine was too apt a comparison for cartoonists to miss. This print is one example, showing Uncle Sam being offered a bottle of "Black Draught Dr. Andrews" by a black boy.

From *Vanity Fair,* Vol. 6, Sept. 6, 1862, p. 119

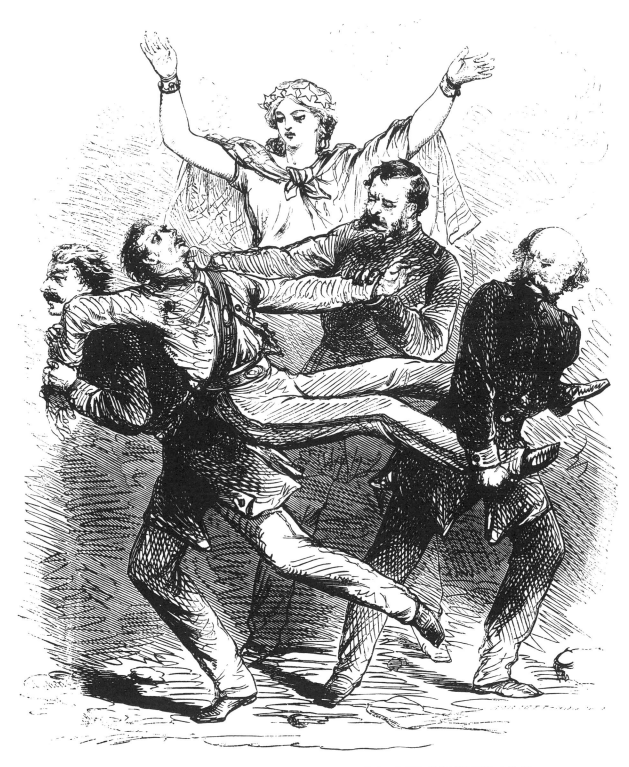

A HINT FOR STATE SURGEON-GENERALS.

Columbia.—"Oh! what a precious lot of Saw-Bones you are! The Wounded Soldier belongs not to this State or that. He belongs to the Union, and I will nurse him!"

64. A Hint for State Surgeon-Generals.
Engraving by H. L. Stephens, 1862.
One of many prints dealing with the rivalry between North and South. This one shows three physicians battling for jurisdiction over a wounded soldier. Columbia admonishes them.

From *Vanity Fair*, Vol. 6, July 5, 1862, p. 7

the social role of the professions

As the physician and pharmacist are traced in prints over the period from the seventeenth century onwards, there is a subtle change in treatment from pomposity to disrespect to neutrality to, most recently, grudging respect. This new respect is founded on the advance of science in the more recent period and the role of the professions as participants in this advance. Since the Renaissance, the doctor and pharmacist have appeared in a variety of different guises, mostly unflattering. One simple reason for this is noted by Dana, "if one were deliberately to hunt for the good that has been said of physicians, it would be found vastly to outweigh the evil, but it would not be as amusing to read...."[13]

In general, we may sum up the tenor of the prints issued in the United States between 1765 and 1870 as showing the physician and pharmacist as inadequate providers of health care to the people. The practitioner is despised for his quackery (e.g., Nos. 13 and 22) and condemned for his avarice (e.g., No. 5). He is even shown haggling over the payment price of a body for dissection (No. 65). Rarely is he depicted in the prints as a respected member of the community. His general appearance, however, is far better than that accorded him in the British prints of the late eighteenth century where he was the subject of derision, scorn and often hate. The anonymous American engraving of *The Election Humbly Inscribed* ...of 1765 reflects the attitudes toward the physician by the caricaturist in this earlier period (No. 23). In any event, both doctor and pharmacist are shown in the political prints in the way the layman viewed them, and the prints "pay attention to the history of the rank and file doctor and the other medical workers"[14] rather than the ideal.

Many of the American medical and pharmaceutical prints issued before 1860 are neutral in their depiction of the social position of the physician and pharmacist. Thus, Paul Revere's two engravings of physicians ministering to America in the 1770's give no indication of the position of the doctor (Nos. 44 and 45). However, later illustrations do offer some comment on the physician's role. D. C. Johnston's *Confab Between John Bull and Brother Jonathan* is bitter in its denunciation of quacks who convinced Brother Jonathan to undergo amputation (No. 22). Uncle Sam also rails at the inadequate treatment he is receiving from doctor, apothecary, and nurse in an 1838 caricature, noting that he was quite hearty "till the Doctor and the rest of you took me in hand" (No. 8). But both of these prints reflect the fact that although treatment by the quacks is poor, there is better help in store from regularly licensed practitioners who perhaps should have been called in from the beginning.

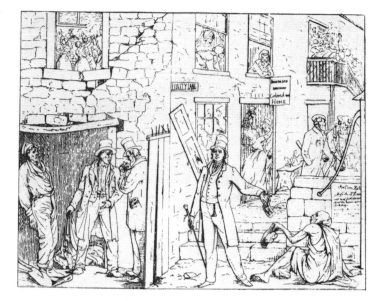

65. Free Negroes in the North. Etching by Adelbert Volck, 1863. A print from the series of *Civil War Etchings* issued by Volck. This is a savage commentary on what evils could be expected to follow from the Emancipation Proclamation; at one side of the print a physician and two blacks are discussing the sale of a body for dissection.

From New York Historical Society

An 1839 caricature of a surgical operation affords some indication of the lack of antiseptic conditions prevailing at that time (No. 14). However, as advances in medicine took place, the political cartoonist was quick to reflect change in his prints as the example of the Letheon shows (No. 30). The sum total of these prints of the pre-Civil War era and earlier, because the number of diseases shown and the drugs used are so few in number, further illustrates the limitations of knowledge and the scope of medicine and pharmacy during the early nineteenth century. The breadth of knowledge did expand during the 1860-1870 decade, as reflected in the prints, but still not significantly.

There is no hint in the total group of any prestigious position being accorded to the profession in the social structure; one could not normally expect this from caricature. At best, the physician and pharmacist are tolerated in the face of the inadequacy of their knowledge. As Leake points out, "The extent and sharpness of the caricature in a particular period depends on the status of the profession and the manner in which it is fulfilling its fundamental obligations to society."[15] The American examples, at least up to 1870, appear, in general, to reflect nothing more than a grudging tolerance.

13. Dana, p. 89
14. Henry E. Sigerist, *A History of Medicine,*
    New York, 1951, Vol. 1, p. 14
15. Leake, p. 2

The prints on this and the following pages, while not specifically discussed in the text, further demonstrate the wide variety of medical and pharmaceutical themes used by political cartoonists during the nation's first century.

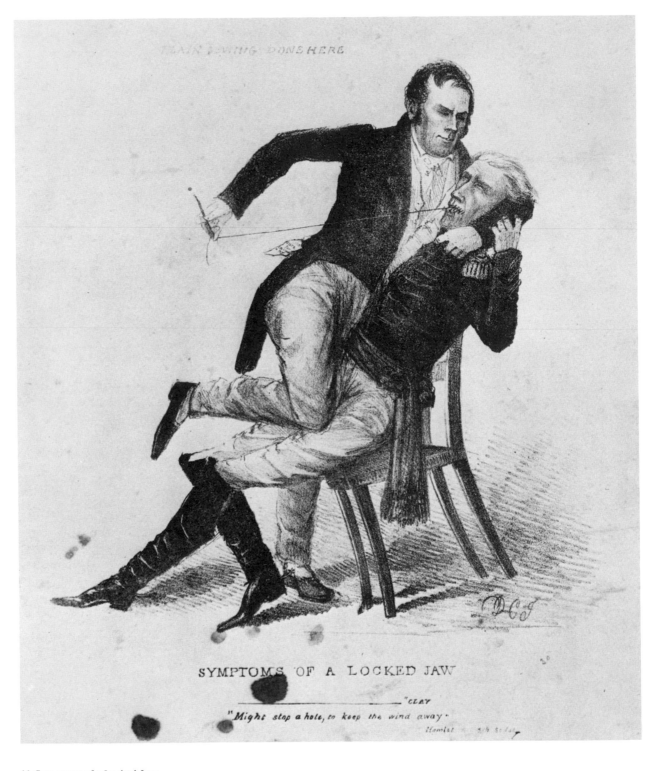

66. Symptoms of a Locked Jaw.
Lithograph by D. C. Johnston, 1834.
A print reflecting the continual differences between Henry Clay and Andrew Jackson, showing the former sewing up Jackson's mouth. In particular, Johnston's effort was issued after Clay had led the Senate to condemn what was felt to be an unwarranted assertion of executive power at the expense of the legislators. The subject of lockjaw also figures in a cartoon of 1861 (see No. 91).

Weitenkampf, p. 34; Butterfield, p. 93, Nevins and Weitenkampf, p. 45; Hess & Kaplan, p. 71; Foreign Policy Assn., p. 17

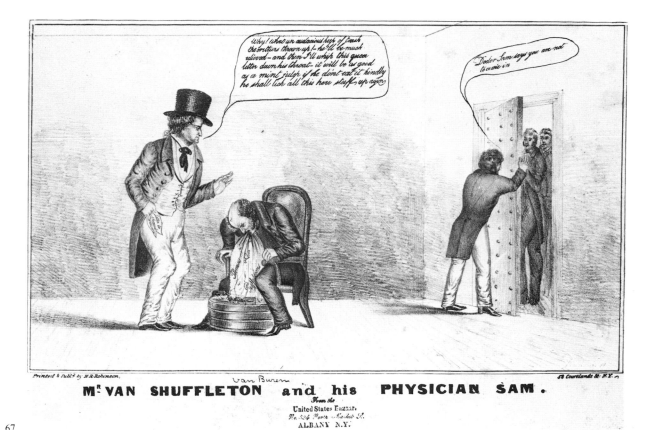

67

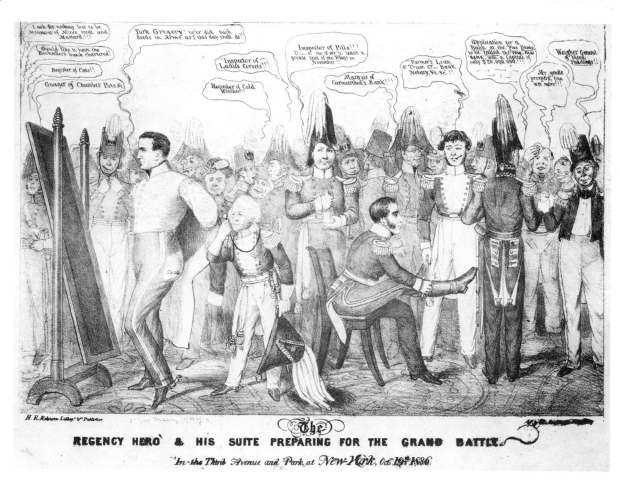

67. Mr. Van Shuffleton and his Physician Sam.
Lithograph by H. R. Robinson, 1836.
This print refers to a letter Van Buren received from Sherrod Williams, a Kentucky member of the House of Representatives, during the campaigning for the election in 1836. The letter asked Van Buren's opinions on a variety of matters, including the distribution of surplus revenues, public land sales, a U.S. Bank, etc. Van Buren is shown vomiting "Promises, Vows, Professions." The physician attending him, Uncle Sam, recommends he "whip this queer letter down his throat—it will be as good as a mint julep."

68. Regency Hero & his Suite Preparing for the Grand Battle....Lithograph by H. R. Robinson, 1836.
A satire on the office seekers in New York appealing to Governor Marcy for jobs. Among them is a man holding a mortar and pestle who wants to be "Inspector of Pills."

Weitenkampf, p. 45

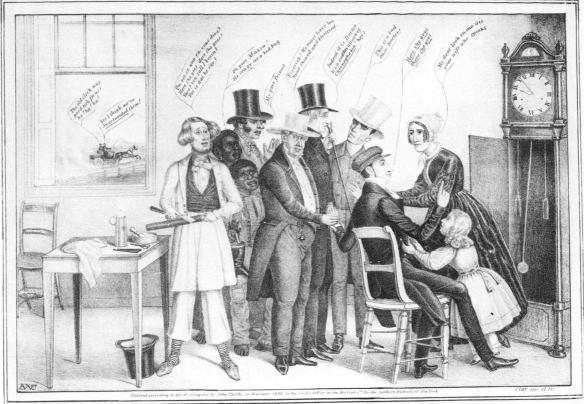

THE OLD CLOCK
Published by J. CHILDS, 119 Fulton St. New York

69. The Old Clock. Lithograph by E. W. Clay, 1838.
A comment on the financial manipulations of a governmental appointee, Samuel Swartwout, in the Van Buren administration. Among a group of people in an office is a doctor taking the pulse of a man seated in a chair. He notes that the patient is "Feverish! We must have his head shaved and blistered." Others present note that the patient has suffered an attack of "Chronophobia." Weitkenkampf, p. 56

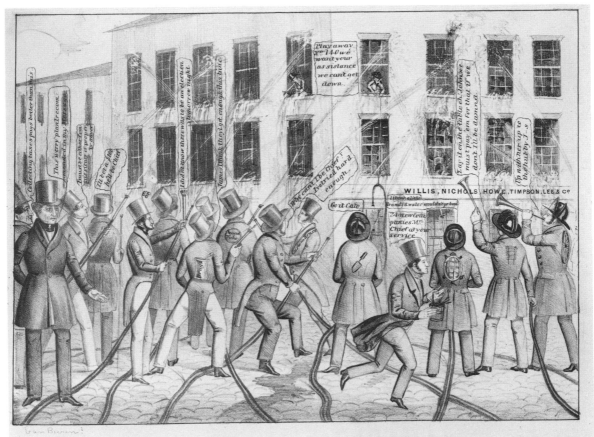

LOCO-FOCOS SQUIRTING
H. R. Robinson's Lith. 52 Courtland. & No 2 Wall St N.Y. 1839

70. Loco-focos Squirting (alternate title: June Bugs Squirting). Lithograph by H. R. Robinson, 1838.
The Loco-focos were a faction of the Democratic Party in New York made up of workingmen and reformers; during Van Buren's administration they controlled party activities in that state. The print shows firemen playing their hoses on a building; one of them is Van Buren, who was allied with the Loco-foco group. Several of the firemen have various symbols on the backs of their uniforms; one has a mortar and pestle and a label "Drugs" on his coat.

Weitkenkampf, p. 52

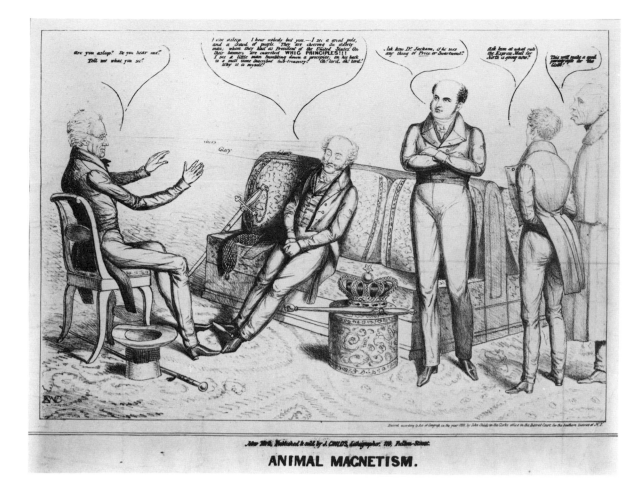

71. Animal Magnetism. Lithograph by E. W. Clay, 1839.
An anti-administration caricature prior to the elections of 1840.
Jackson, as a hypnotist, is mesmerizing the patient, President
Van Buren.

Weitenkampf, p. 58

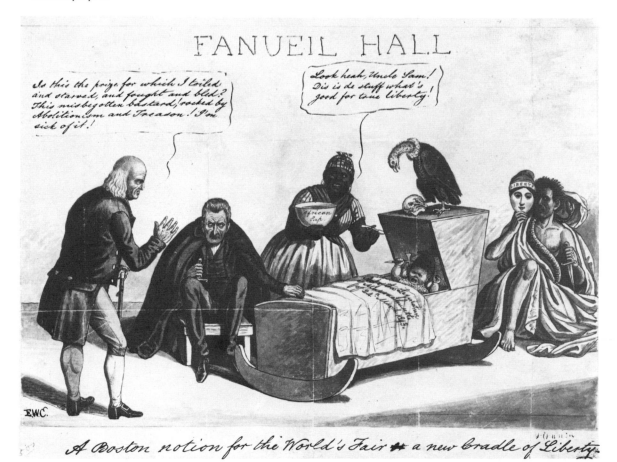

72. A Boston notion for the World's Fair—a new Cradle of
Liberty. Drawing by E. W. Clay, 1843.
One of the early graphic comments on the slavery question. A
nurse is shown ready to administer some "African Pap" to an
infant in a cradle while Uncle Sam looks on.

Weitenkampf, p. 72

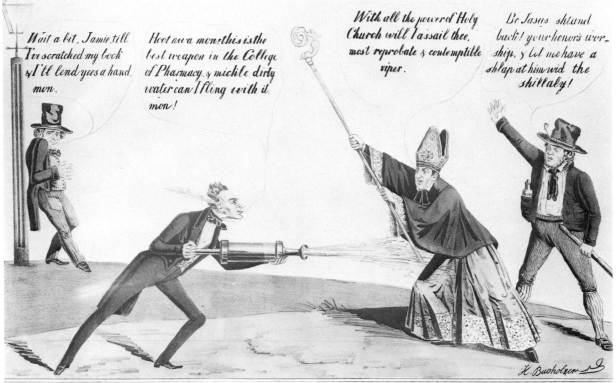

73. Jamie & the Bishop. Lithograph by H. Bucholzer, 1844.
A graphic comment on political differences between James
Gordon Bennett, the editor, and Archbishop Hughes of New
York. Bennett squirts the preparation in a large clyster at the
Archbishop, saying "Hoot awa mon, this is the best weapon in
the College of Pharmacy."

Weitenkampf, p. 83

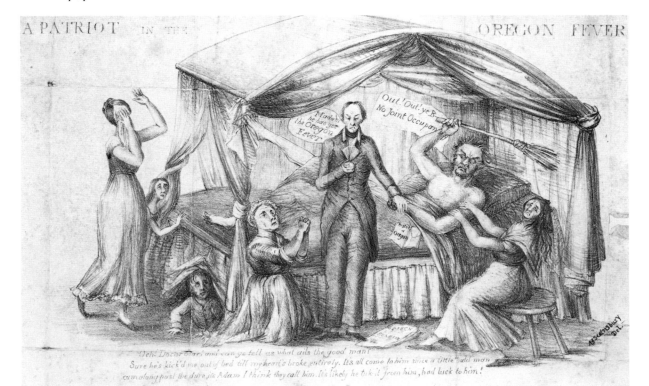

74. A Patriot in the Oregon Fever.
Lithograph by A. Scansbury, 1844.
This print deals with problems between the United States and
England over the Oregon Territory. A doctor, feeling the pulse
of the patient, notes "Madam he has got the Oregon fever."
The patient screams "Out! Out! ye B_____.
No joint occupancy."

Weitenkampf, p. 77

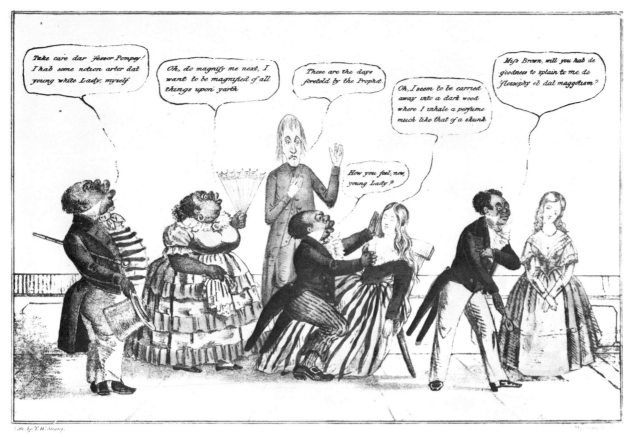

PROFESSOR POMPEY MAGNETIZING AN ABOLITION LADY.

75. Professor Pompey Magnetizing an Abolition Lady.
Lithograph by T. W. Strong, 1845.
A humorous comment on the efforts of the abolitionists
to eliminate slavery. The print shows a group of blacks
and whites, with one of the former group hypnotizing
a white woman.

Weitenkampf, p. 85

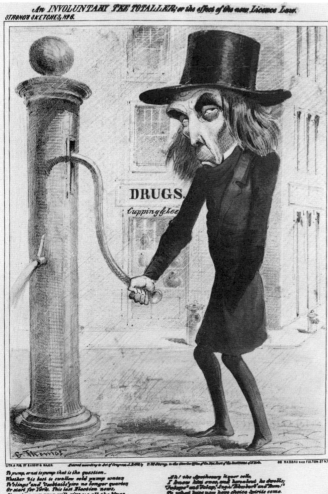

76. An Involuntary Tee Totaller; or the effect of the new
Licence Law. Lithograph by G. Thomas, 1846.
A satire on the elections of 1846 and temperance activities
in New York. A drunkard is shown at a pump; in the
background is a storefront with a sign "Drugs. Cupping
& Lee...." The verse is a parody on Hamlet's soliloquy.

Weitenkampf, p. 87

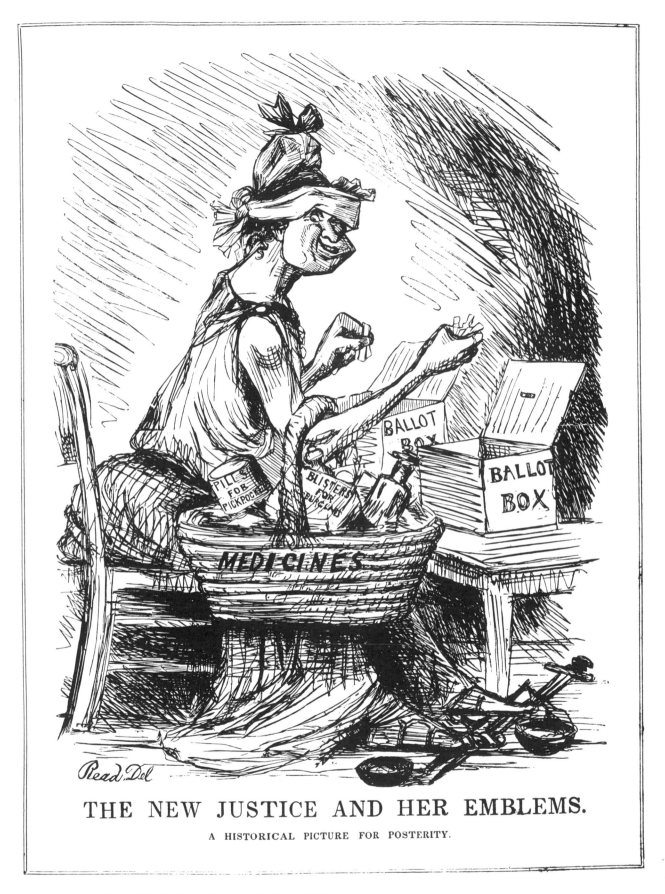

THE NEW JUSTICE AND HER EMBLEMS.

A HISTORICAL PICTURE FOR POSTERITY.

77. The New Justice and Her Emblems. Engraving by Read, 1847.
A cartoon suggesting various solutions for several problems with
which the Polk administration had to deal. A seated woman
holds a basket of "Medicines" in which are "Blisters for Burglars,"
"Pills for Pickpockets," etc.

From *Yankee Doodle*, Vol. 2, 1847, p. 105

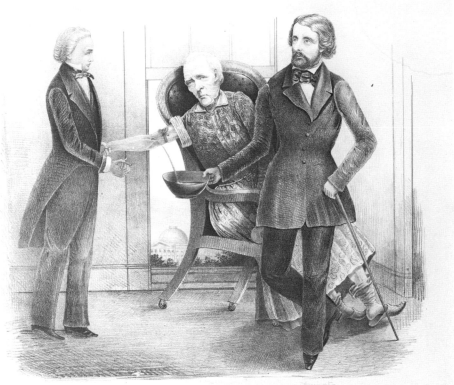

LETTING THE LAST "*DEMOCRATIC DROP*"

78. Letting the Last "Democratic Drop."
Anonymous lithograph, c. 1856.
The election of 1856 was between James Buchanan and John C.
Fremont. The print shows two physicians bleeding the patient,
the Democrat Buchanan. One of the physicians is Fremont.

From American Antiquarian Society

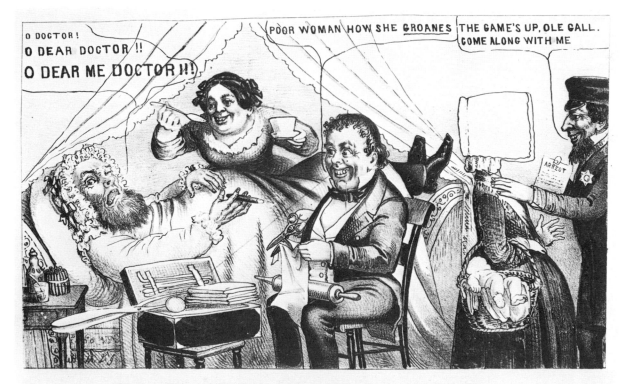

MRS CUNNINGHAM AND HER BLESSED BABY

Published at 46 Arch St

79. Mrs. Cunningham and her Blessed Baby.
Anonymous lithograph, 1857.
A satire on a notorious murder in New York City in which the
wife of Dr. Burdell, a Mrs. Cunningham, was the accused in a
widely publicized murder trial. The patient is a bearded
Cunningham, attended by a doctor with a scissors and clyster.

A box of his surgical implements is nearby. A nurse, holding a cup
and spoon is also present, and there is a glass of medicine ready
for the patient as well.

From Library Company of Philadelphia

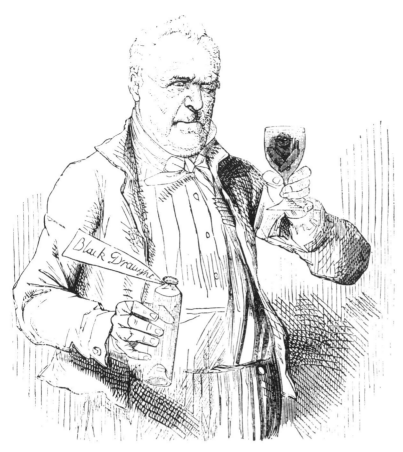

MR. BUCHANAN TASTING THE DRINKING WATER AT WASHINGTON.
FROM "PUNCH."

80. Mr. Buchanan Tasting the Drinking Water at Washington. Anonymous engraving, 1857.
Perhaps the most important domestic crisis of the Buchanan administration was the slavery question, a subject alluded to in this cartoon, which appeared earlier in the British humor weekly, *Punch*. It shows President Buchanan drinking from a goblet in which is a black boy. The President holds in his right hand the bottle from which his medicine was taken; it is labeled "Black Draught."

From *Frank Leslie's Illustrated Newspaper*, Vol. 3, April 11, 1857, p. 293

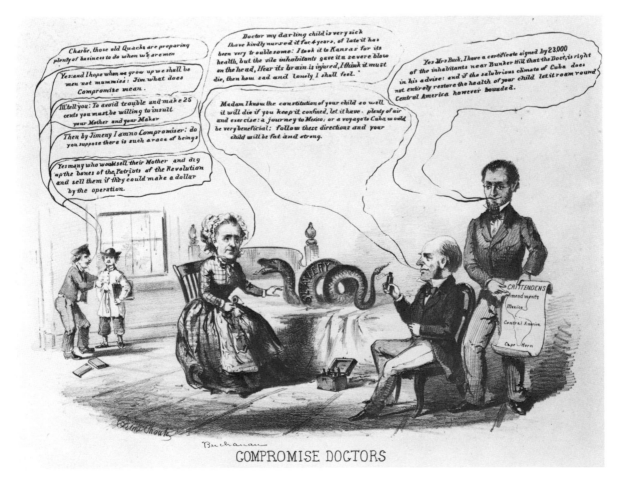

COMPROMISE DOCTORS

81. Compromise Doctors. Anonymous lithograph, 1860.
The Crittenden Compromise was an unsuccessful attempt to prevent secession. This print is a graphic comment on it, showing physicians attending a patient, in this case a snake labeled "Slavery." The patient's mother is Buchanan; one of the doctors is Crittenden, who holds a bottle of medicine. At his feet is a box of other medicines. A boy comments "...those old quacks are preparing plenty of business to do when we are men."

Weitenkampf, p. 120

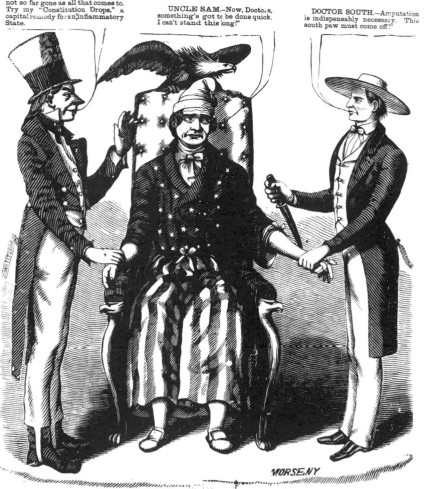

82. North and South Treating Uncle Sam. Wood engraving by F. Morse, 1860.
A print commenting on the sectional differences prior to the election of 1860. Two doctors are shown attending Uncle Sam; Dr. North recommends, "Try my 'Constitution Drops'," noting that they are "a capital remedy for an inflammatory State." Dr. South feels that "Amputation is indispensably necessary."

Weitenkampf, p. 125

"SICH A GITTIN UP STAIRS."

"Miss Douglas heller out. Den she jump between us
But i guess she so forgit de day wen Abra'm show his genus!
Sich a gittin up stairs i neber did see.
Sich a gittin up stars i neber did see!"

83. "Sich A Gittin Up Stairs." Engraving by H. L. Stephens, 1860.
Another of the candidates competing with Lincoln was John C. Breckenridge. In this print he is shown fighting with Lincoln; both are presented as physicians, as their stethoscopes indicate.

From *Vanity Fair*, Vol. 2, Oct. 27, 1860, p. 213; Wilson, p. 71

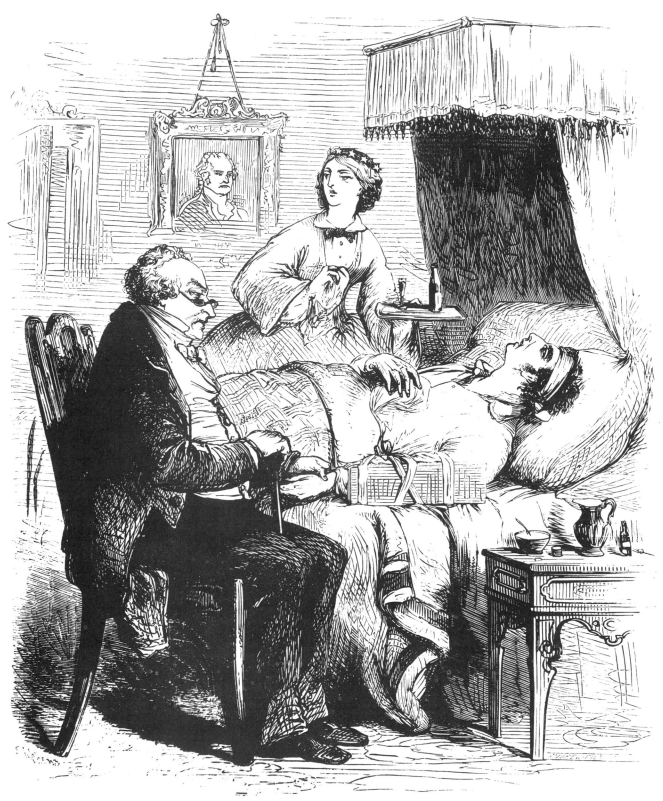

BROTHER JONATHAN LAME.

Doctor Disunion.—Poor Fellow! His constitution is so run down that I fear he cannot survive without an amputation.
Nurse Columbia.—O! *don't* give it up, Doctor. Good nursing will do anything—everything—if you will only give him the opportunity.

84. Brother Jonathan Lame. Engraving by H. L. Stephens, 1860.
Stephens' cartoon refers to the burning question of the day—the
survival of the Union. The print shows a physician (Doctor
Disunion), a nurse (Columbia) and a sick patient (Brother
Jonathan). The recumbent patient has his arm in a sling, and
some of his medicines are nearby.

From *Vanity Fair*, Vol. 2, Dec. 8, 1860, p. 285; Shaw, p. 151

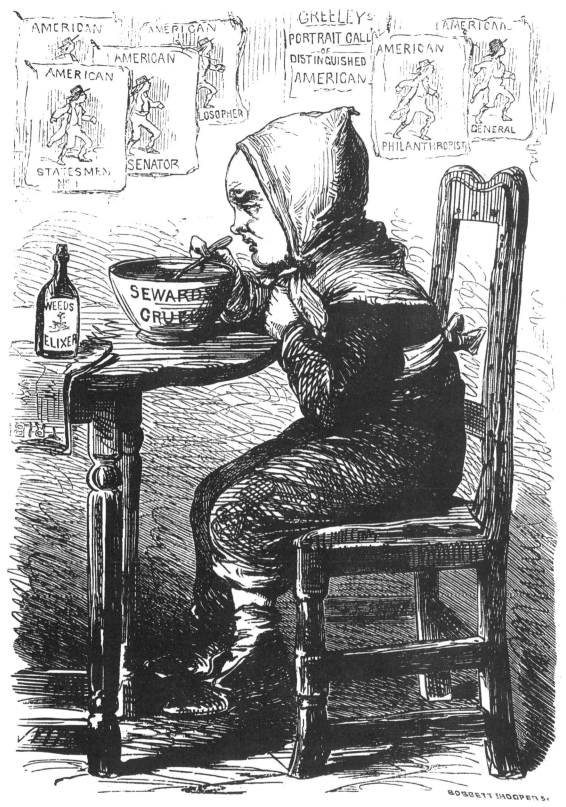

HORACE SICK!

Poor Boy! well give him his Gruel and Elixir. He'll soon be up and round as saucy as ever!

85. Horace Sick! Anonymous engraving, 1861.
Greeley, the editor of the New York Tribune, was miffed after
Lincoln's election, in that Senator Seward and Thurlow Weed
were of greater influence on the President than he was. The
cartoon shows Greeley at a kitchen table on which are "Weeds
Elixer" and "Sewards Gruel," which should cause him to recover
quickly.

From *Vanity Fair*, Vol. 3, Feb. 16, 1861, p. 78; Shaw, p. 213

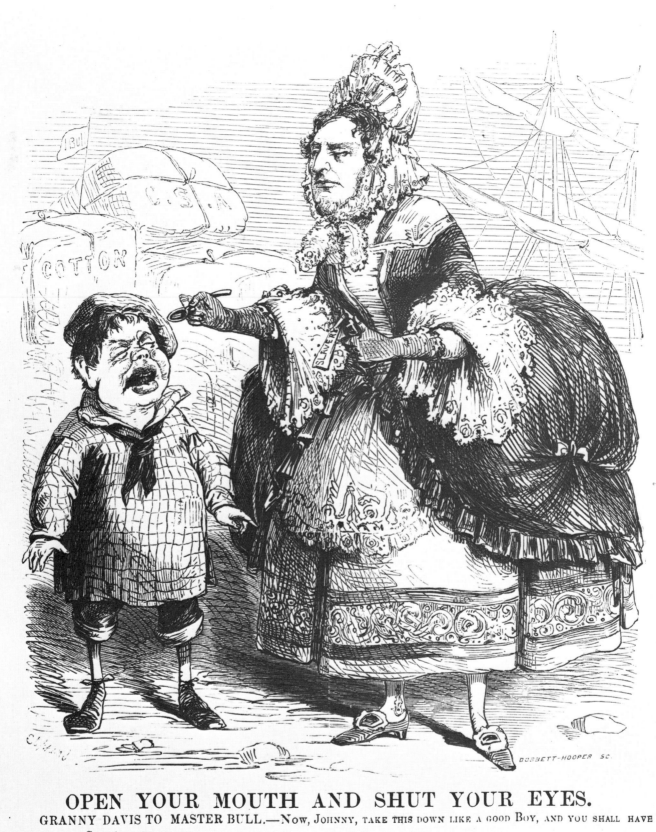

OPEN YOUR MOUTH AND SHUT YOUR EYES.

GRANNY DAVIS TO MASTER BULL.—Now, JOHNNY, TAKE THIS DOWN LIKE A GOOD BOY, AND YOU SHALL HAVE AS MUCH NICE COTTON AS YOU WANT.

86. Open Your Mouth and Shut Your Eyes. Engraving by
H. L. Stephens, 1861.
A cartoon commenting on the cotton trade between England and
the South. Jefferson Davis is shown giving medicine from a bottle
labeled "Slavery" to a crying John Bull.

From *Vanity Fair*, Vol. 3, Mar. 30, 1861, p. 151

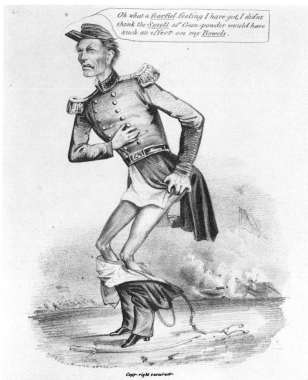

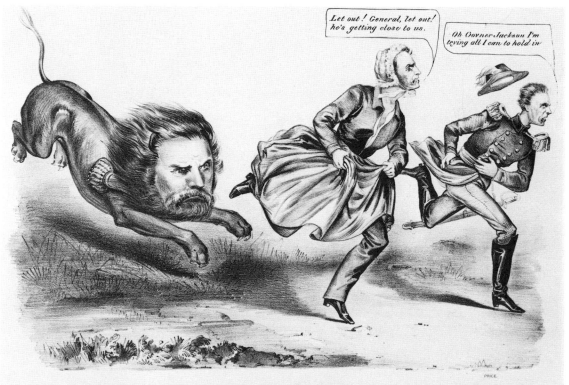

87. Battle of Booneville, Missouri, June 18th, 1861.
Anonymous lithograph, 1861.
Several of the prints illustrating aspects of the
Civil War have some medical interest as does
this one of the confederate general, Stirling Price,
with an attack of diarrhea (See Nos. 88, 92, 55).

Weitenkampf, p. 130

88. The Battle of Booneville, or the Great Missouri "Lyon" Hunt.
Anonymous lithograph, 1861.
Another print with the same subject as the previous one. Here
the northern general, Nathaniel Lyon, chases two "Rebel"
generals, Claiborne F. Jackson and Stirling Price (See Nos. 87,
92, 55).

Weitenkampf, p. 130

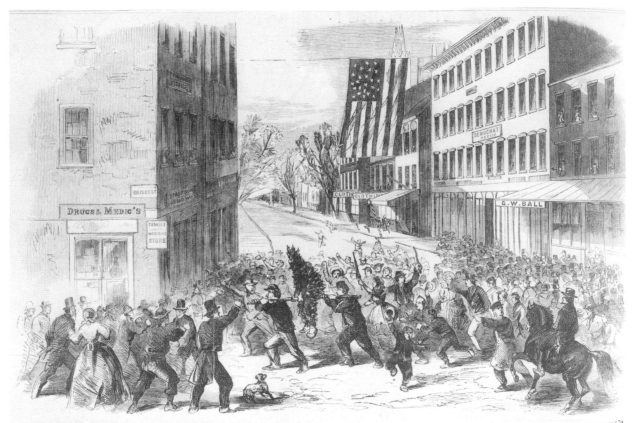

TARRING AND FEATHERING OF AMBROSE L. KIMBALL, EDITOR OF THE ESSEX "DEMOCRAT," HAVERHILL, MASS., A REBEL-SYMPATHISING JOURNAL.—FROM A SKETCH BY A CORRESPONDENT.—SEE PAGE 259.

89. Tarring and Feathering of Ambrose L. Kimball, Editor of the Essex "Democrat," Haverhill, Mass. A Rebel-Sympathising Journal. Anonymous engraving, 1861.
Kimball "…had sorely tried the loyalty and patience of the community by his violent articles in favor of Secession," according to the text of an article that accompanied this illustration, and the result was not too pleasant for him. The mob surrounding Kimball appears in front of some buildings near a street corner; one of these is a pharmacy with signs reading "Family Medicine Store" and "Drugs & Medic's."
From *Frank Leslie's Illustrated Newspaper*, Vol. 12, Aug. 31, 1861, p. 256

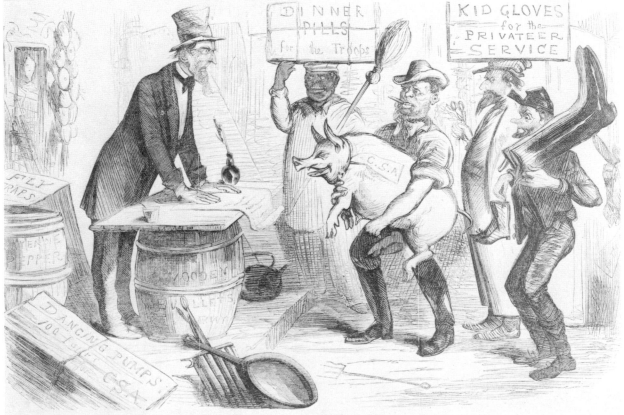

JEFF AT THE RECEIPT OF CUSTOMS; OR, SOUTHERN TAXES BEING PAID IN KIND.

90. Jeff at the Receipt of Customs; or, Southern Taxes Being Paid in Kind. Anonymous engraving, 1861.
A print issued to satirize the inability of the government of the southern states to raise needed revenue. It shows Jefferson Davis accepting goods being offered to him; one of the items presented is a box of "Dinner Pills."
From *Frank Leslie's Illustrated Newspaper*, Vol. 12, Oct. 12, 1861, p. 352

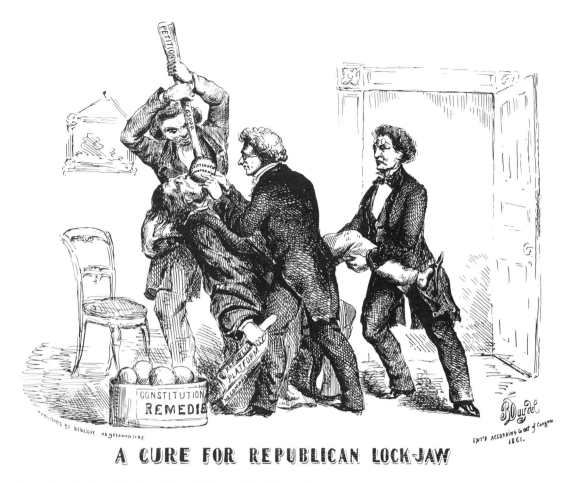

A CURE FOR REPUBLICAN LOCK-JAW

91. A Cure for Republican Lock-Jaw. Lithograph by B. Day, 1861.
A caricature on the Crittenden Compromise, showing three Democrats attempting to force it down the throat of a patient. One holds the pill labeled "Crittenden Compromise," while a second stamps it down with a club labeled "Petition of 63,000." The pill had been taken from a box marked "Constitution[al] Remedie[s]."

Weitenkampf, p. 130; Shaw, p. 153; Dannett, p. 21

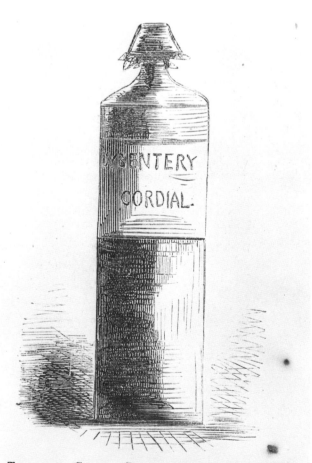

THE REBEL GENERAL PRICE ALWAYS TRAVELS WITH A STRONG BODY GUARD, AT LEAST SO STATE THE REBEL NEWS-PAPERS. WE BEG LEAVE TO OFFER A "BODY GUARD" THAT THE GENERAL SHOULD NEVER BE WITHOUT.

92. Dysentery Cordial. Anonymous engraving, 1862.
Another satire on General Price and his gastrointestinal problems (Nos. 87, 88, 55). The cartoon offers the bottle of medicine as a " 'body guard' that the general should never be without."

From *Yankee Notions*, Vol. 11, Jan., 1862, p. 10

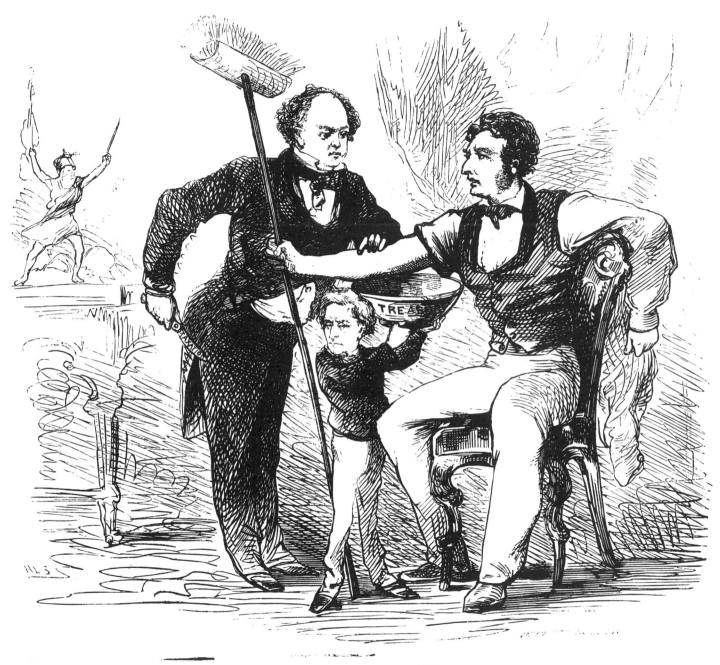

THE GOOD PATIENT.

Uncle Sam.—" WELL, DR. CHASE, IF YOU MUST BLEED ME WHY DON'T YOU BEGIN?

93. The Good Patient. Engraving by H. L. Stephens, 1862.
This cartoon reflects Union financial difficulties during the Civil War.
It shows Salmon P. Chase, the Secretary of the Treasury, ready to bleed
Uncle Sam for more money; the cup in which the blood will be received
is labeled "Treasury," and the lancet Chase holds is labeled "Taxation."

From *Vanity Fair*, Vol. 5, Jan. 25, 1862, p. 41

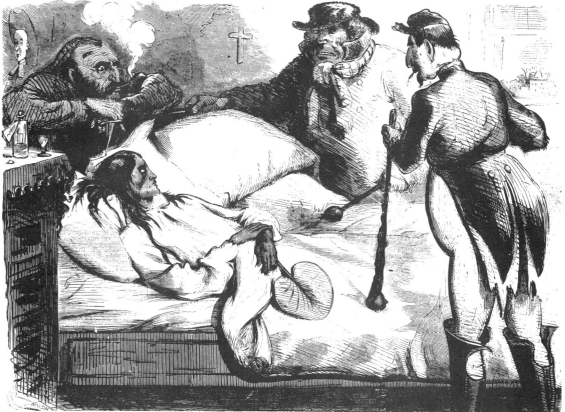

THE SICK WOMAN OF MEXICO.——JOHN BULL. "Say, Missus! me and these other Gents 'ave come to Nurse you a bit."

94. The Sick Woman of Mexico, Engraving by Frank Bellew, 1862.
A graphic comment on the interest certain European nations were showing in Mexico during the time of the Civil War. Mexico is symbolized as a patient in bed, as three men, representing France, England and Spain, look on. The patient's medicine is on a table next to her bed.

From *Harper's Weekly*, Vol. 6, Feb. 8, 1862, p. 96

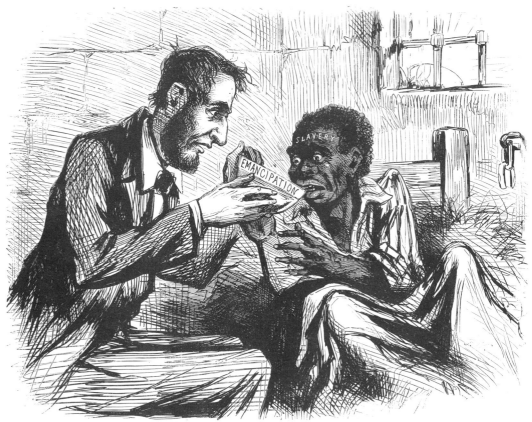

DOCTOR LINCOLN'S NEW ELIXIR OF LIFE—FOR THE SOUTHERN STATES.

95. Doctor Lincoln's New Elixir of Life—For the Southern States.
Wood engraving by Thomas Nast, 1862.
Although the Emancipation Proclamation was not finally issued until 1863, there was much discussion of it in the previous year. Nast's cartoon deals with the question, showing Lincoln giving a dose of "emancipation" to a black boy.

From the *New York Illustrated News*, Vol. 5, April 12, 1862, p. 368

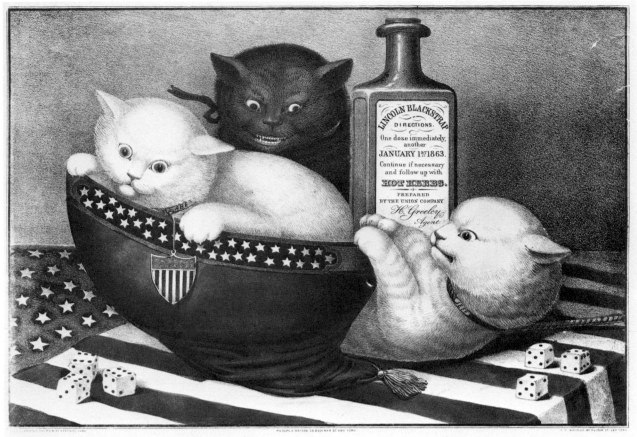

96. The Great Remedy. Anonymous lithograph, 1862.
The Emancipation Proclamation is pictured as "The Great Remedy" in this print. Three cats are playing on a flag on which is a large bottle of medicine, "Lincoln Blackstrap."

Weitenkampf, p. 135; Nevins & Weitenkampf, p. 98.

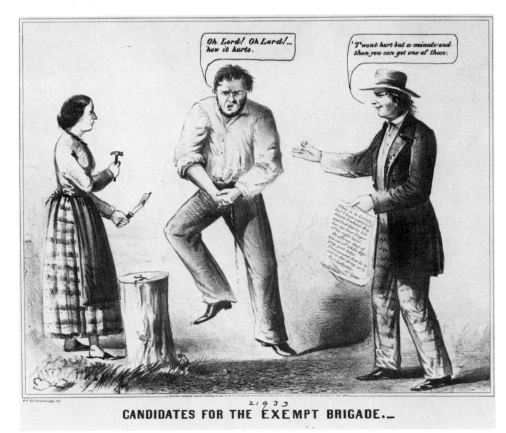

97. Candidates for the Exempt Brigade. Lithograph by Wm. F. S. Trowbridge, c. 1862.
As is usually the case with a draft of manpower in times of war, there are many men anxious to avoid conscription. This print reflects this desire; it shows a man who has just had part of his finger chopped off by his wife or sweetheart. A friend holds a certificate signed by a physician in order to exempt him from service as a result of his loss.

From Library of Congress

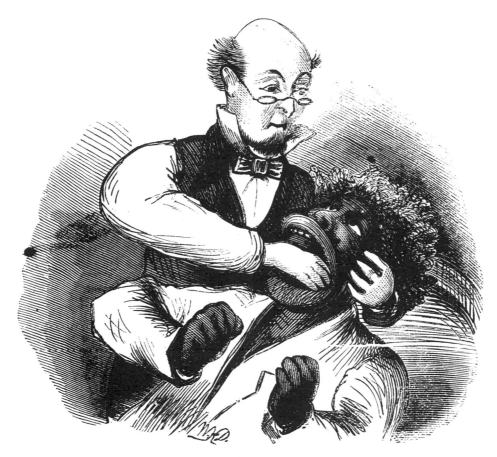

Getting his Hand In.

98. Getting his Hand in. Anonymous engraving, 1863.
Horace Greeley is portrayed as a dentist, with his hand in the mouth
of a black man, about to pull a tooth. The print is a reference to Greeley's
attempts to influence the government in regard to the war effort.

From *Yankee Notions*, Vol. 12, January, 1863, p. 14

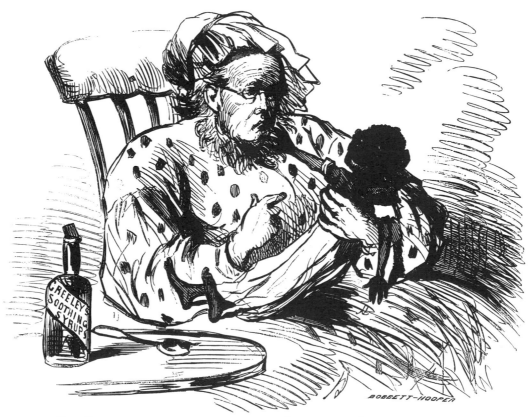

NURSE GREELEY HARDLY KNOWS WHAT TO THINK ABOUT BABY, NOW: IT ISN'T SUCH A BEAUTY, AFTER ALL.

99. Nurse Greeley hardly knows what to think about Baby, now;
it isn't such a beauty, after all. Anonymous engraving, 1863.
An anti-Greeley satire, showing him as a nurse, holding a small black
baby. Nearby is a bottle of "Greeleys Soothing Syrups."

From *Vanity Fair*, Vol. 7, Jan., 1863, p. 8

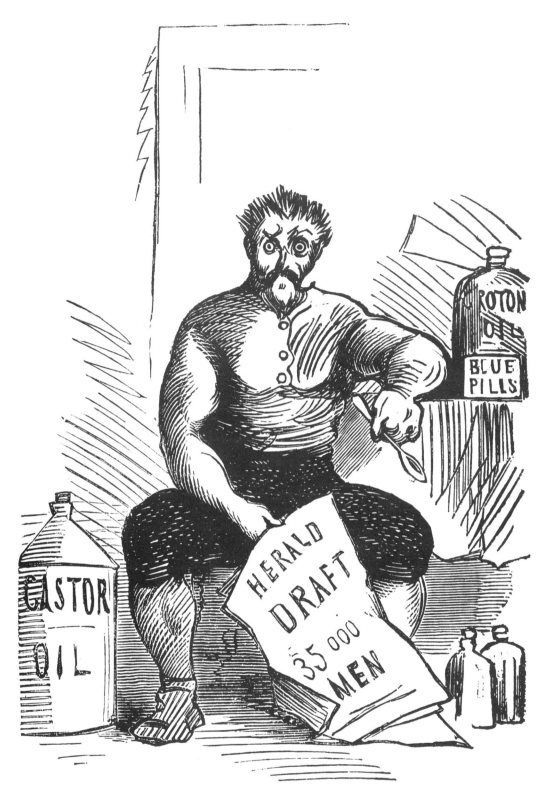

POWERFUL EFFECT OF THE LATE ACCOUNT OF THE MILL IN ENGLAND, ON KNOCK-EM-STIFF. NEEDS FURTHER CONSIDERATION BEFORE HE HAS HIS TURRET TRIED. THINKS HE'LL REDUCE HIMSELF, AND TRY IT SOME OTHER TIME.

100. Powerful effect of the late account of the mill in England, on Knock-em-stiff. Anonymous engraving, 1863.
A cartoon on draft evasion. A strong man is shown holding a paper on which is printed "Herald Draft 35,000 men." Some medicines are nearby. The print is a companion to one showing the subject when he was more concerned with building his strength, rather than tearing it down.

From *Yankee Notions*, Vol. 12, Feb., 1863, p. 43

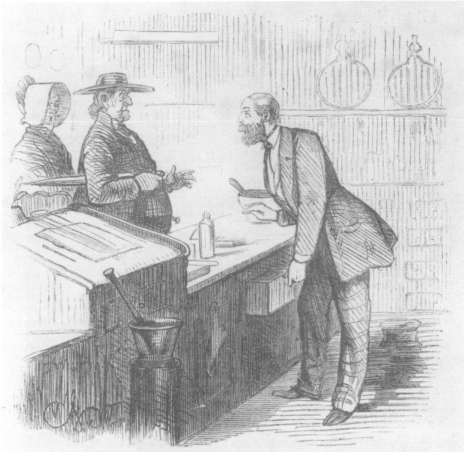

THE CURRENCY QUESTION—MAKING CHANGE.

STOREKEEPER—"*I've no pennies—would you mind taking a ticket for the Broadway 'Free and Easy" instead?*"

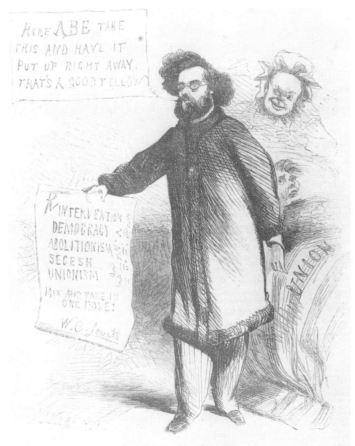

"ENOUGH TO KILL HIM."

The Colorado grand Peace Prescription.

101. The Currency Question—Making Change. Engraving by William Newman, 1863.
A comment on the financial pressures the North was undergoing during the middle of the Civil War.

From *Frank Leslie's Illustrated Newspaper*, Vol. 15, Mar. 14, 1863, p. 400

102. "Enough to Kill Him." Engraving by Ward, 1863.
The many proposals for ending the war are illustrated in this cartoon which is subtitled "The Colorado grand Peace Prescription." Holding his prescription is William Cornell Jewett of Colorado, a friend of Horace Greeley and a prolific correspondent to both northern and southern leaders in vain attempts to bring peace. He addresses Lincoln, advising him to "…take this and have it put up right away…." His prescription calls for:

Intervention	1 oz.
Democracy	2 oz.
Abolitionism	2 oz.
Secesh	2½ oz.
Unionism	2 oz.

From *Frank Leslie's Illustrated Newspaper*, Vol. 16, March 28, 1863, p. 16

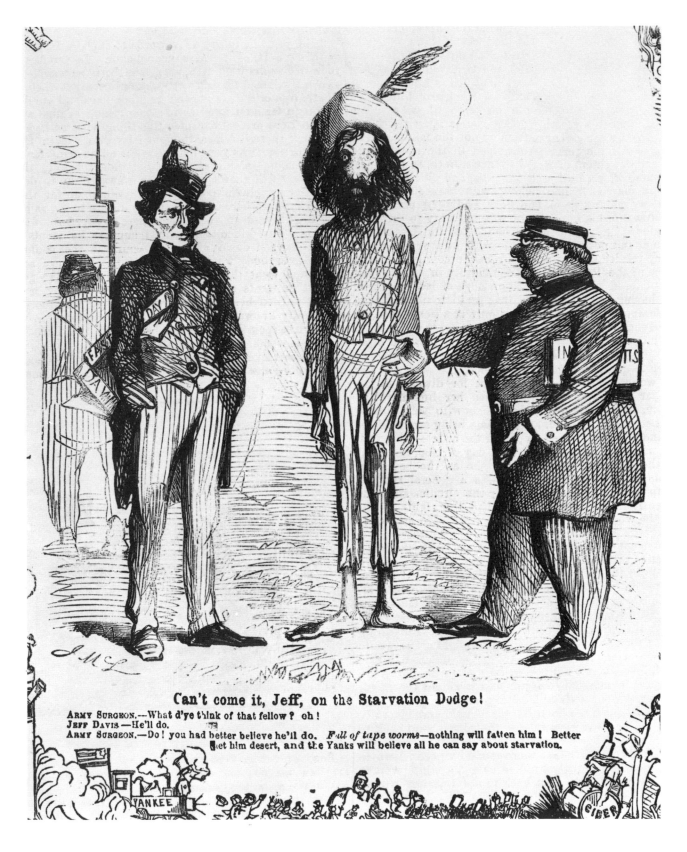

103. Can't come it, Jeff, on the Starvation Dodge.
Anonymous engraving, 1863.
A satirical comment on the problems of the South in getting enough
rations for their troops. Three men, an Army surgeon, Jefferson
Davis, and a soldier with worms stand together. The surgeon suggests
that the soldier desert so that the enemy will believe what he will
say about starvation.

From *Yankee Notions*, Vol. 12, June, 1863, p. 161

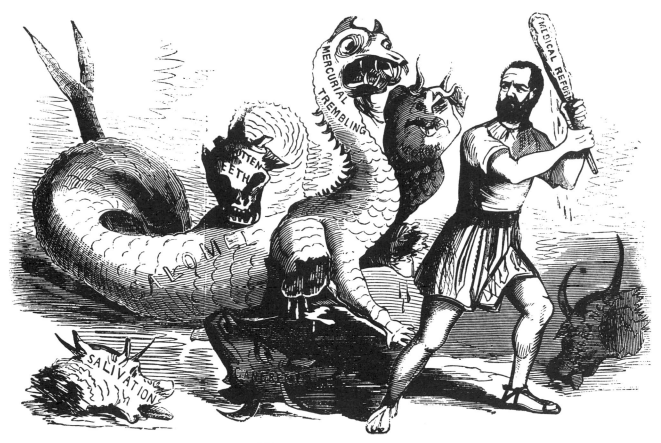

THE MODERN HERCULES.

Surgeon-General Hammond crushing out the Hydra Calomel.

104. The Modern Hercules. Anonymous engraving, 1863.
An illustration of the efforts of the Surgeon General of the
Union Army, William A. Hammond, to reduce the usage of
calomel by the physicians in the army by removing it from the
supply table. Hammond is shown wielding a club labeled
"Medical Reform," as he attacks "Gangrene," "Salivation,"
"Mercurial Trembling," "Rotten Teeth," etc. These are all parts of
the Hydra "Calomel," the basic source of all the difficulty.

From *Frank Leslie's Illustrated Newspaper*, Vol. 16, Aug. 1, 1863,
p. 308

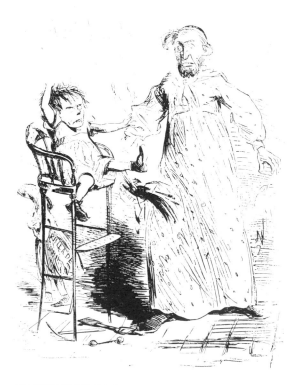

THE NAUGHTY BOY GOTHAM, WHO WOULD NOT TAKE THE DRAFT.

MAMMY LINCOLN—*"There now, you bad boy, acting that way, when your little sister Penn takes hers like a lady!"*

105. The Naughty Boy Gotham, Who Would Not Take the Draft.
Anonymous engraving, 1863.
Another print on the draft riots, this one again using the
draft/draught theme. It shows Lincoln, as a nurse, rebuffed by
a little boy in a high chair, who tosses over a bowl of "Draft."

From *Frank Leslie's Illustrated Newspaper*, Vol. 16, Aug. 29, 1863,
p. 372; Wilson, p. 245

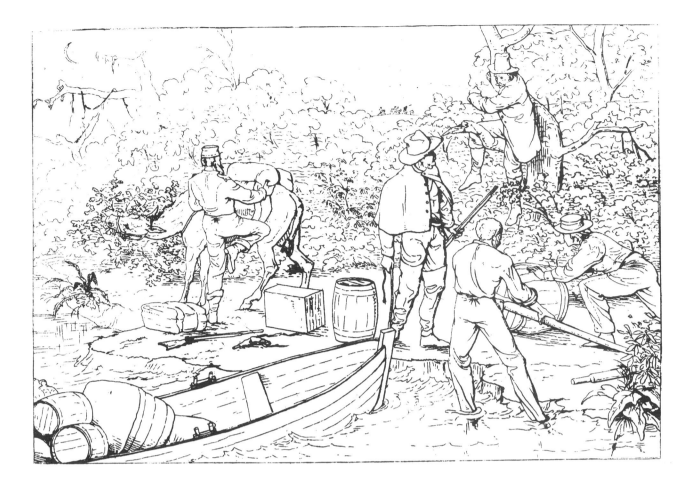

106. Smuggling Medicines into the South.
Etching by Adelbert Volck, 1863.
Volck, a practicing dentist, was one of the few artists to issue
political prints for the Confederate side during the Civil War.
Of the 30 plates in his set of etchings, two have some medical
overtones, this one and No. 65. Here a group of men are
shown removing boxes of medicines from a boat; one in a
tree serves as a lookout for enemy forces.

From Countway Library of Medicine

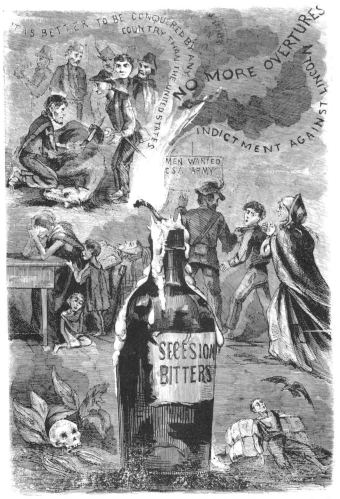

107. The Last Ditch; or, the Death Struggles of the
Southern Confederacy. Anonymous engraving, 1864.
By spring, 1864, the Southern forces were in deep trouble, as
this cartoon notes. It shows a large bottle of "Secession
Bitters" giving off fumes with various labels, "Indictment
against Lincoln," etc.

From the *New York Illustrated News*, Vol. 9, March 12, 1864,
p. 305

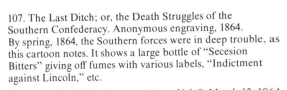

THE LAST DITCH: OR, THE DEATH-STRUGGLES OF THE SOUTHERN CONFEDERACY.

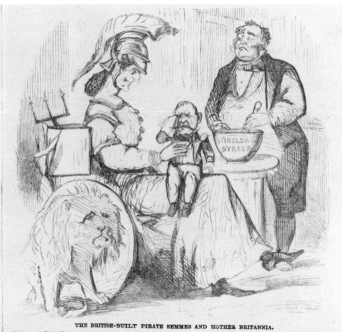

THE BRITISH-BUILT PIRATE SEMMES AND MOTHER BRITANNIA.

BRIT.—"*Did the nasty, lanky Yankee sink his pretty, itty ship! Never mind, then—his mammy shall build him another, she shall. Don't he cry then ——*" *etc.*—See London *Times* and other English journals.

108. The British-Built Pirate Semmes and Mother Britannia. Anonymous engraving, 1864.
This print is a satire on the sinking of the Confederate pirate ship, Alabama, captained by Raphael Semmes, by the Union ship, the Kearsarge, under Captain Winslow. John Bull is shown stirring some "Winslow Syrup" with a pestle as Semmes, portrayed as a sick child, laments his loss. The Alabama had been built in England and was sold to the Confederacy.

From *Frank Leslie's Illustrated Newspaper,* Vol. 18, July 23, 1864, p. 228

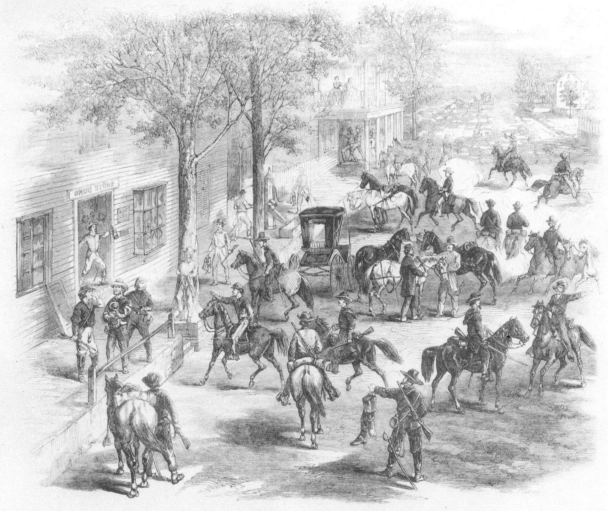

THE RAID INTO MARYLAND.—REBEL CAVALRY OCCUPYING THE TOWN OF NEW WINDSOR.—FROM A SKETCH BY FREDERICK DIELMAN.

109. The Raid into Maryland—Rebel Cavalry Occupying the Town of New Windsor. Engraving after Frederick Dielman, 1864.
An illustration of military activity during the latter part of the Civil War. Troops are shown in front of a drug store, in the windows of which can be seen several show globes.

From *Frank Leslie's Illustrated Newspaper,* Vol. 18, Sept. 3, 1864, p. 381

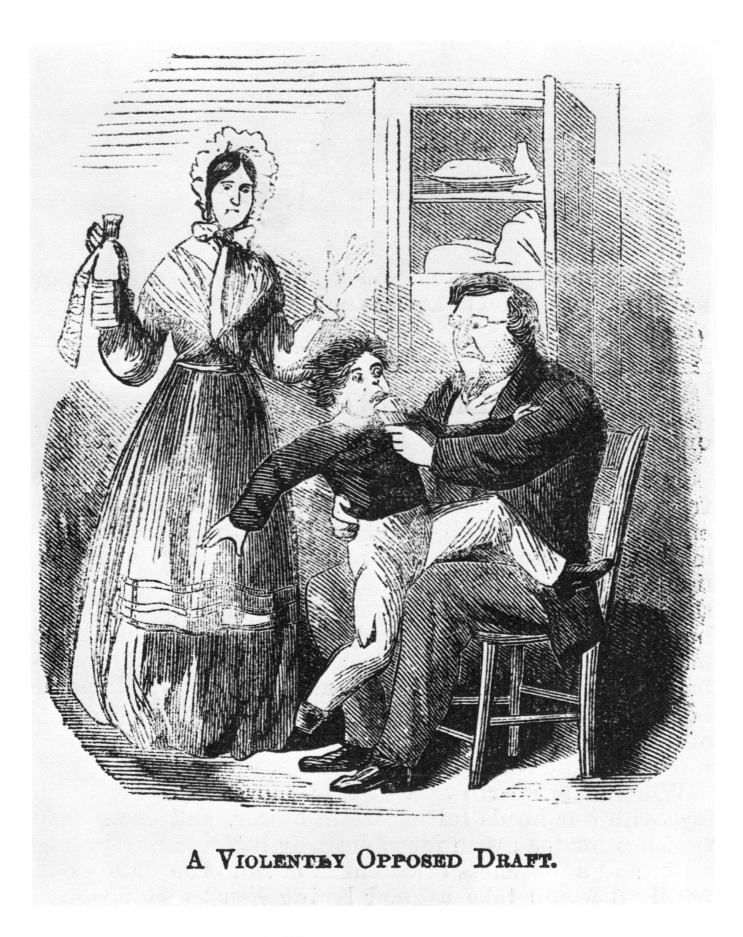

A VIOLENTLY OPPOSED DRAFT.

110. A Violently Opposed Draft. Anonymous engraving, 1864.
One illustration of several designed to accompany an article
entitled "The Draft." This one shows a physician giving
medicine to a boy; his mother watches, holding a bottle of
medicine labeled "Castor Oil."

From *Yankee Notions*, Vol. 13, October, 1864, p. 313

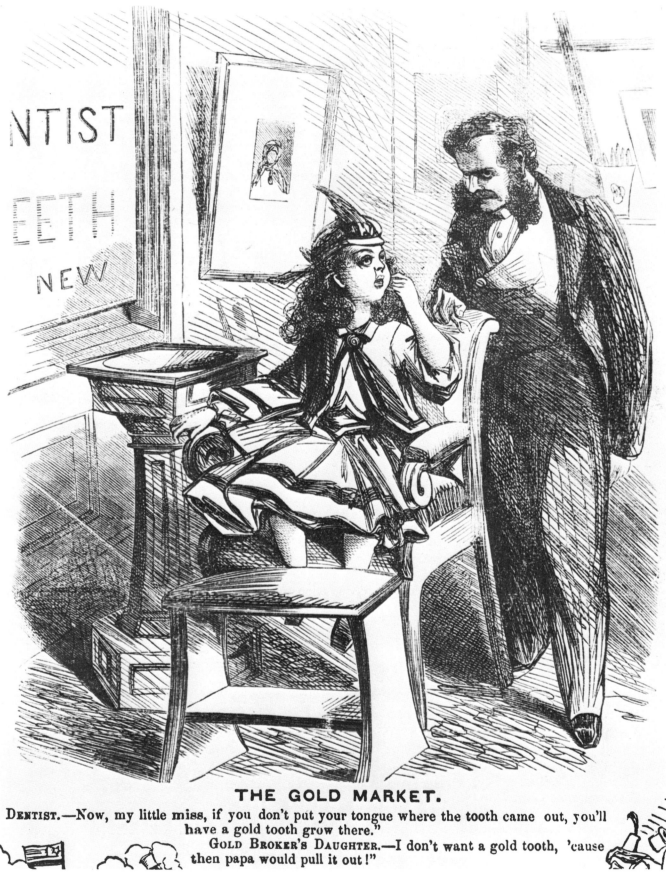

THE GOLD MARKET.

DENTIST.—Now, my little miss, if you don't put your tongue where the tooth came out, you'll have a gold tooth grow there."

GOLD BROKER'S DAUGHTER.—I don't want a gold tooth, 'cause then papa would pull it out!"

111. The Gold Market. Engraving by Howard, 1865.
Economic conditions at the close of war forced the price of gold
up; this cartoon alludes to this problem. It shows a dentist
talking to a girl in his chair; he asks her to move her tongue so
that he can put in a new gold tooth. But, as the gold broker's
daughter, she is afraid her father will remove it because of its value.

From *Yankee Notions*, Vol. 14, August, 1865, p. 225.

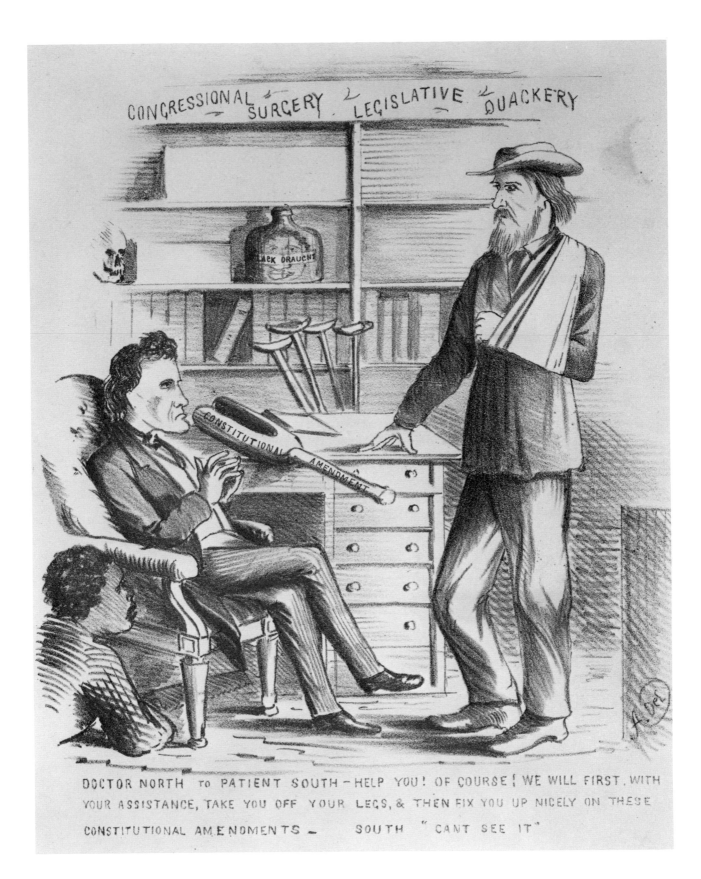

112. Congressional Surgery Legislative Quackery.
Anonymous lithograph, 1866.
A print discussing reconstruction efforts at the War's end. A
doctor, President Johnson, is shown at a desk behind which is a
bottle of "Black Draught"; he addresses a southerner with a
bandaged arm.

Weitenkampf, p. 153

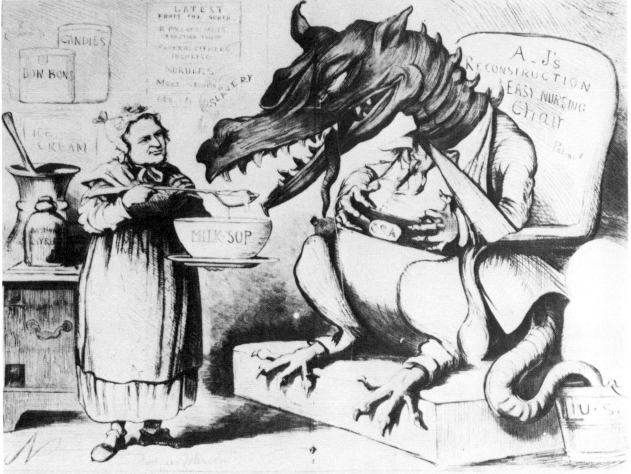

OUR EXECUTIVE FEEDING UP THE SOUTHERN DRAGON

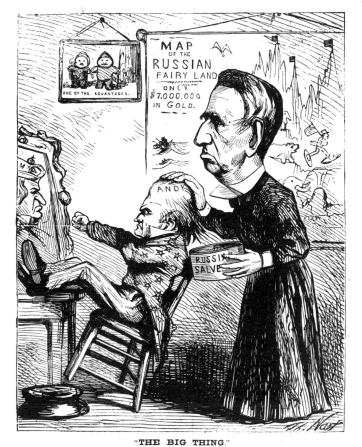

"THE BIG THING."

OLD MOTHER SEWARD. "I'll rub some of this on his sore spot; it may soothe him a little."

113. Our Executive Feeding Up the Southern Dragon. Lithograph by William Newman, 1866.

Johnson's conciliatory policy toward the defeated South is the subject of this caricature. It shows the President, as a nurse, offering "milk sop" to a grotesque dragon, representing the Confederate States. Other bottles, jars, and a mortar and pestle are also shown.

From *Frank Leslie's Budget of Fun*, 1866; Murrell II, pp. 6-7.

114. "The Big Thing." Engraving by Thomas Nast, 1867. This cartoon has the purchase of Alaska by William H. Seward as its subject. Seward is shown applying some "Russian Salve" to the bald head of President Johnson.

From *Harper's Weekly*, Vol. 11, April 20, 1867, p. 256

73

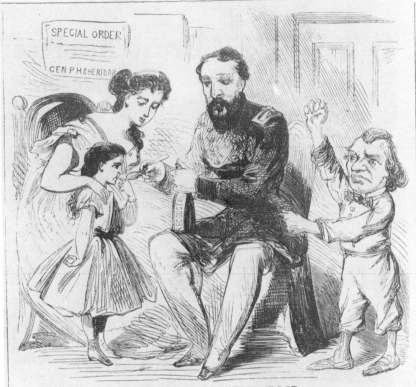

THE RECONSTRUCTION DOSE.

NAUGHTY ANDY—" *Don't take that physic, Sis, it's nasty—kick his shins.*"
MRS. COLUMBIA—" *My dear Andy, don't be a bad boy, don't interfere—Dr. Congress knows what's best for Sissy.*"

115. The Reconstruction Dose. Anonymous engraving, 1867.
A cartoon on the problems of reconstruction after the War was over. A doctor, representing Congress, is shown administering some "Reconstruction" medicine to a little girl, held by Columbia. Andrew Johnson is the little girl's brother, who warns her not to take the medicine.

From *Frank Leslie's Illustrated Newspaper,* Vol. 24, July 13, 1867, p. 272

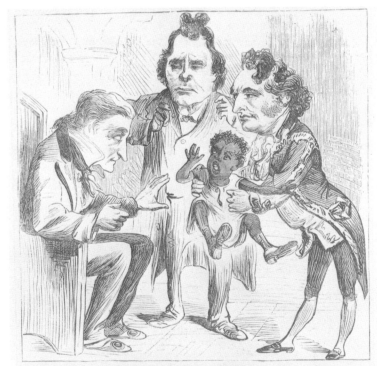

TOO BLACK A DOSE.

DR. SUMNER—" *My dear Uncle Sam, Dr. Stevens and myself are quite convinced that the only way to reconstruct your health is to swallow this dear little darkey whole.*"
DR. THAD STEVENS—" *It's easily done—it's only to open your mouth very wide—he is not much bigger than a good-sized oyster.*"
UNCLE SAM—" *You mean well, my boys, no doubt. I have swallowed an Irishman and a Dutchman, and don't feel much the worse, but that nigger would be the death of me.*"

116. Too Black a Dose. Anonymous engraving, 1867.
A cartoon comment on Reconstruction. Charles Sumner and Thaddeus Stevens are depicted as physicians; they offer their patient, Uncle Sam, as medicine, a black boy, recommending he swallow it. But Uncle Sam refuses, noting that he has "...swallowed an Irishman and a Dutchman, and don't feel much the worse...."

From *Frank Leslie's Illustrated Newspaper,* Vol. 25, Nov. 23, 1867, p. 160

THE BOTTLE IMP!

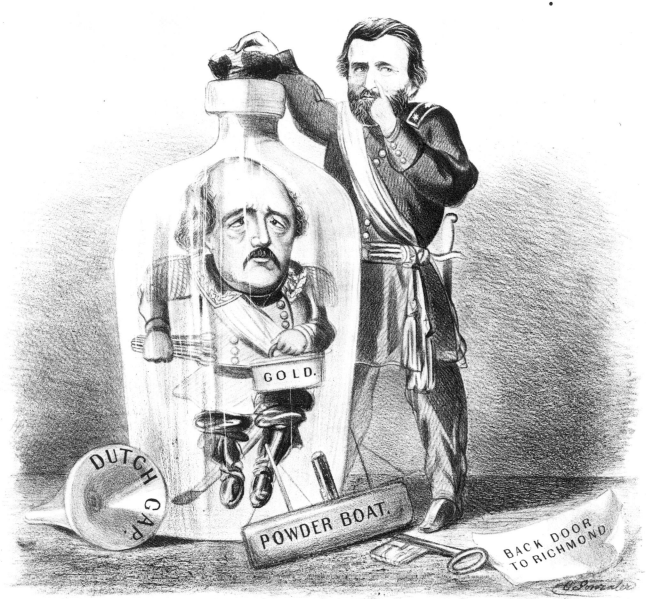

GOLD.

DUTCH GAP.

POWER BOAT.

BACK DOOR TO RICHMOND

PUB.BY.WM.C.ROBERTSON 59 CEDAR ST NY.

LOWELL BITTERS BOTTLED BY GRANT.
B. F. B. 1865 — U. S. G.

117. The Bottle Imp! Lithograph by E. Gonzalez, 1868. General Benjamin F. Butler, at the time of this caricature, was a Representative in Congress from Massachusetts. Although a member of Grant's Republican party, there were some differences of opinion regarding Grant's nomination for the Presidency, which this print illustrates. Grant is shown with his hand on the top of a large bottle of "Lowell Bitters," with Butler, holding the spoons with which he was usually associated, inside.

Weitenkampf, p. 157

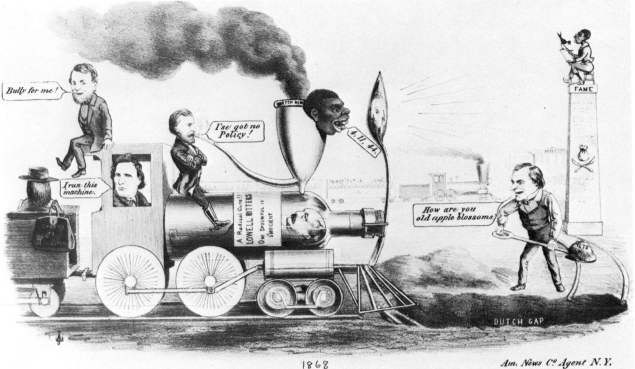

FATE OF THE RADICAL PARTY.

118. Fate of the Radical Party. Anonymous lithograph, 1868.
A second print dealing with Grant and Butler. This one shows
Grant sitting on a locomotive, the main part of which is a bottle
labeled "Lowell Bitters," as the train heads for the Dutch Gap.

An inscription on the bottle reads "A Radical Cure!!
Lowell Bitters— one spoonful is sufficient."

Weitenkampf, p. 157.

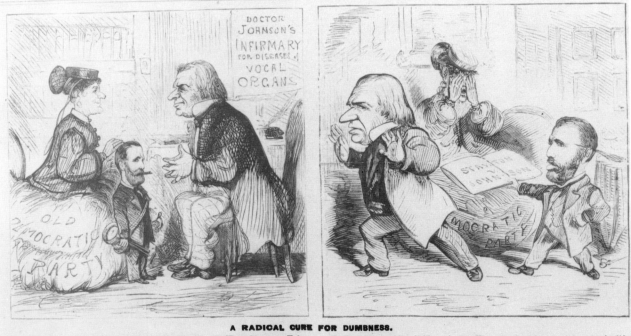

A RADICAL CURE FOR DUMBNESS.

ANXIOUS OLD LADY—"Dear Doctor, there's something the matter with Ulysses' tongue. He has not spoken for six months."
DOCTOR—"Ha! yes, I see; we'll soon cure him of that."

The Doctor's treatment works like a miracle. Ulysses speaks right out, and astonishes the Old Lady and Doctor with a couple of naughty valentines.

119. A Radical Cure for Dumbness. Anonymous engraving, 1868.
Grant's influence on national politics was substantial even before
the nominating conventions of 1868. At the time of this cartoon
President Johnson was facing impeachment proceedings and had
just dismissed Edwin M. Stanton, the Secretary of War, and had
appointed Grant in his place. Two scenes are shown in the print,
the first in a doctor's office with the physician, Johnson, attending

a mother (the "Old Democratic Party") and her son, Grant. A sign
on the wall reads "Doctor Johnson's Infirmary for Diseases of
Vocal Organs." In the second cartoon, Grant holds a paper
labeled "Stanton v. Johnson," and frightens both the mother and
the doctor.,

From *Frank Leslie's Illustrated Newspaper*, Vol. 25, Feb. 29, 1968,
p. 384

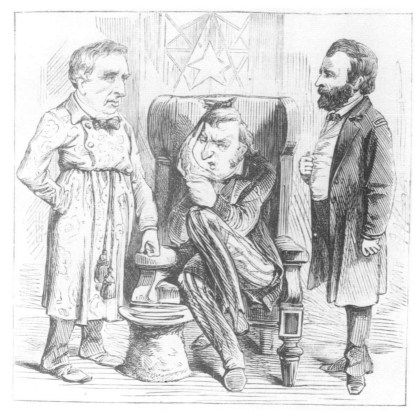

UNCLE SAM'S BAD TOOTH—THE ANDY JOHNSON GRINDER.

DR. GRANT—"*I say, out with it at once. He'll have no peace with it in.*"
DR. SEWARD—"*I'm in favor of letting it stop till it drops out quietly.*"

120. Uncle Sam's Bad Tooth—The Andy Johnson Grinder.
Anonymous engraving, 1868.
The impeachment proceedings against Andrew Johnson were being held in the Senate at the time of this cartoon. It shows Johnson with a frightful toothache, between two doctors, Grant and William H. Seward, both then members of Johnson's cabinet. The physicians debate the preferred treatment.

From *Frank Leslie's Illustrated Newspaper*, Vol. 26, April 25, 1868, p. 96

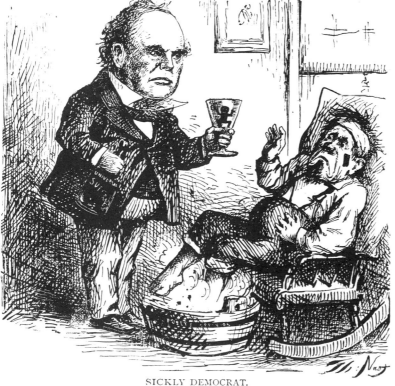

SICKLY DEMOCRAT.
"Oh! must I Swallow him Whole, Doctor Chase?"

121. Sickly Democrat. Engraving by Thomas Nast, 1868.
An election print offered by the consistently pro-Republican cartoonist, Thomas Nast. It shows Salmon P. Chase, who had just finished presiding over the impeachment hearings on Andrew Johnson, offering some advice to the Democratic party—that they should accept the defeat of the recent war more gracefully. Chase offers the patient a glass of medicine in which is a black baby, but the patient is reluctant to take it.

From *Harper's Weekly*, Vol. 12, July 11, 1868, p. 439

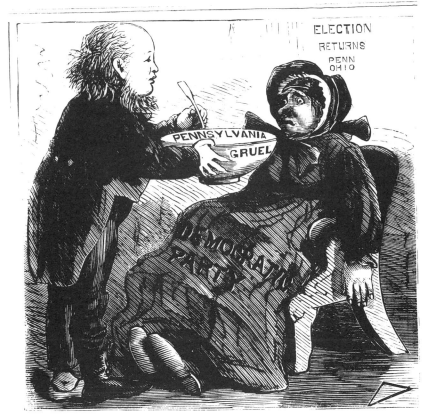

THE OLD DEMOCRATIC PARTY GETS HER GRUEL.

H——G—— "*Now, then, you poor old creature, take this and go to bed quietly. As you've got to die, you may as well do it decently.*"

122. The Old Democratic Party Gets her Gruel.
Engraving by Frank Bellew, 1868.
An election print for 1868, when Grant was the Republican candidate and Horatio Seymour the Democratic. Horace Greeley, who was to be the Liberal-Democratic candidate four years later,

is shown offering a sick woman (the "Democratic Party") a bowl of "Pennsylvania Gruel."

From *Frank Leslie's Illustrated Newspaper*, Vol. 27, Oct. 31, 1868, p. 112

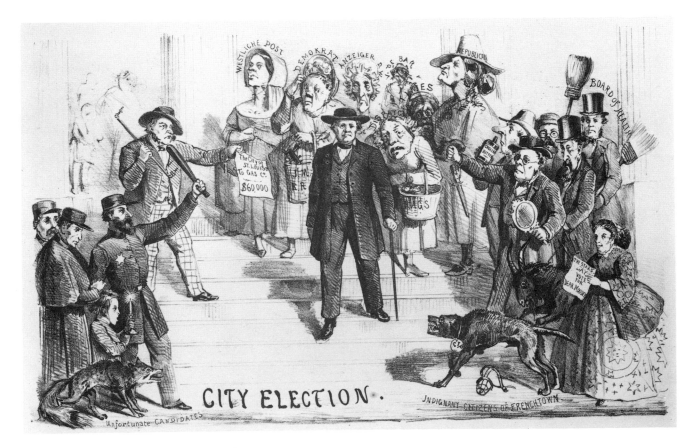

123. City Election. Anonymous lithograph, 1869.
A graphic comment on a local election in St. Louis. The print includes a group of men from the "Board of Health," one of whom drinks from a bottle of "Cholera Bitters."

Weitenkampf, p. 161

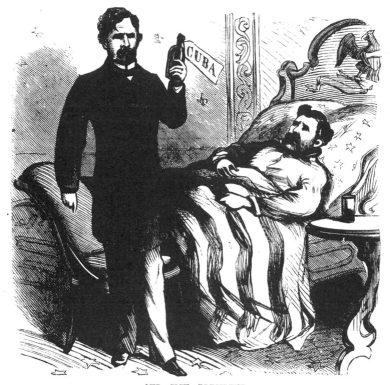

OUR SICK PRESIDENT.

DR. BANKS.—"*Ah! Um! Too much Fish—too much Fish. Eh? Hum! Fever! Take a little of this!*"

124. Our Sick President. Anonymous engraving, 1870. A commentary on the problem with Cuba in Grant's first administration. A physician holds a bottle of medicine labeled "Cuba" as he addresses the patient, President Grant, who lies in bed. He diagnoses the case as having been due to too much fish, a reference to Hamilton Fish, a member of the Grant cabinet. From *Frank Leslie's Illustrated Newspaper*, Vol. 30, July 9, 1870, p. 272

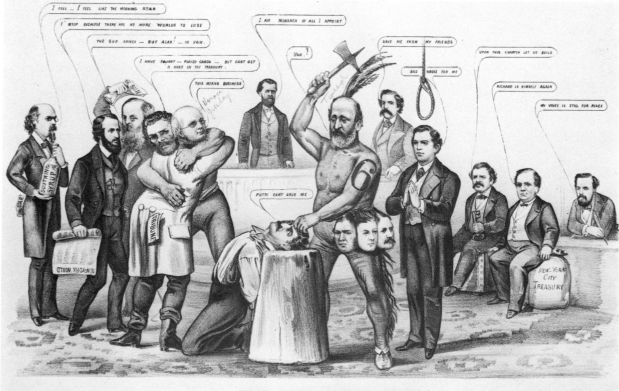

THE JACK KNIFE WAR

125. The Jack Knife War. Anonymous lithograph, 1870. One of the many cartoons, the most significant of which were by Thomas Nast, attacking the Tweed Ring in New York. This print shows a group of men, one of whom is Joe Howard, a newspaper owner, who holds a bottle of "Soothing Syrup." Weitenkampf, p. 162

chronological listing of american political prints of medical and pharmaceutical interest

1765	The Election Humbly Inscrib'd to the Saturday-Nights Club, in Lodge Alley.	**No. 23**
1774	The able Doctor, or America Swallowing the Bitter Draught. Engraving by Paul Revere.	**No. 44**
1775	America in Distress. Engraving by Paul Revere.	**No. 45**
1813	Brother Jonathan Administering a Salutary Cordial to John Bull. Engraving by Amos Doolittle.	**No. 61**
	Queen Charlotte and Johnny Bull Got Their Dose of Perry. Engraving by William Charles.	**No. 62**
1820	A case of infectious fever, (from "81 South Street, No. 62, 4 doors down from Callowhill Street," Philadelphia), before the New York Board of Health. Anonymous engraving.	**No. 6**
1833	The Doctors Puzzled or the Desperate Case of Mother U.S. Bank. Anonymous lithograph.	**No. 5**
	Troubled Treasures. Lithograph by E. Bisbee.	**No. 9**
	Troubled Treasures. Lithograph by R. Bisbee.	**No. 10**
1834	Uncle Sam in Danger. Anonymous lithograph.	**No. 13**
	Symptoms of a Locked Jaw. Lithograph by D. C. Johnston.	**No. 66**
1836	Confab between John Bull and Brother Jonathan. Lithograph by D. C. Johnston.	**No. 22**
	Mr. Van Shuffleton and his Physician Sam. Lithograph by H. R. Robinson.	**No. 67**
	Regency Hero and his Suite Preparing for the Grand Battle. Lithograph by H. R. Robinson.	**No. 68**
1838	Uncle Sam Sick with La Grippe. Lithograph by H. R. Robinson.	**No. 8**
	The Old Clock. Lithograph by E. W. Clay.	**No. 69**
	Loco-Focos Squirting (alternate title: June Bugs Squirting). Lithograph by H. R. Robinson.	**No. 70**
1839	Professor Wise, Performing a Surgical Operation in Congress Hall. Lithograph by H. R. Robinson.	**No. 14**
	Animal Magnetism. Lithograph by E. W. Clay.	**No. 71**
1840	The death of Locofocoism. Anonymous lithograph.	**No. 3**
1843	A Boston notion for the World's Fair—a new Cradle of Liberty. Drawing by E. W. Clay.	**No. 72**
1844	Coroners Inquest on Loco-Focoism. Lithograph by H. Bucholzer.	**No. 4**
	Dose-The-Boys' Hall. Anonymous lithograph.	**No. 24**
	Jamie & the Bishop. Lithograph by H. Bucholzer.	**No. 73**
	A Patriot in the Oregon Fever. Lithograph by A. Scansbury.	**No. 74**
1845	Professor Pompey Magnetizing an Abolition Lady. Lithograph by T. W. Strong.	**No. 75**
1846	An Involuntary Tee Totaller; or the effect of the new Licence Law. Lithograph by G. Thomas.	**No. 76**
1847	Triumph of the Letheon. Anonymous engraving.	**No. 30**
	The Constitution and its Nurses. Anonymous lithograph.	**No. 47**
	The New Justice and Her Emblems. Engraving by Read.	**No. 77**
1848	The Candidate of Many Parties. Lithograph by H. R. Robinson.	**No. 21**
1852	Fighting and Fainting. Anonymous lithograph.	**No. 26**
	The Follies of the Age, Vive la Humbug!! Anonymous lithograph.	**No. 40**
1856	Letting the Last "Democratic Drop." Anonymous lithograph.	**No. 78**
1857	Mrs. Cunningham and her Blessed Baby. Anonymous lithograph.	**No. 79**
	Mr. Buchanan Tasting the Drinking Water at Washington. Anonymous engraving.	**No. 80**
1858	Take the Hint ye who owe Doctor's Bills. Anonymous engraving.	**No. 31**
1860	The Political Invalid. Engraving by H. L. Stephens.	**No. 11**
	Wonderful Surgical Operation. Engraving by H. L. Stephens.	**No. 15**
	The Two Sick Men. Engraving by John Leech.	**No. 46**
	Compromise Doctors. Anonymous lithograph.	**No. 81**
	North and South Treating Uncle Sam. Wood engraving by F. Morse.	**No. 82**
	"Sich a Gittin up Stairs." Engraving by H. L. Stephens.	**No. 83**

civil war envelopes

In both the Northern and Southern states, envelopes and other stationery were used for propaganda purposes during the war period. These began at the very outbreak of the war as patriotic statements, with illustrations of flags, states and portraits of statesmen; later they developed into more vitriolic designs with slogans, mottoes and illustrations that sometimes became rather crude. In most cases the message, either as picture or words or both, took up about a third of the entire envelope, but there are examples of graphic design that cover the entire space, leaving no room for the address.

Although the total number of envelope designs is unknown, several of them had some medical or pharmaceutical interest, usually in the form of political cartoons. They reinforce our understanding of the bitter fanaticism that existed on both sides of the conflict, and also show something of the pervasiveness of medical and quasi-medical concepts at the time. The following is a list of these envelopes. Each of the following was printed in the North.

references

J. S. Bassett, *Makers of a New Nation.*
"The Pageant of America" Series, Vol. 9,
New Haven, Connecticut, Yale University Press, 1928.

C. S. Brigham, *Paul Revere's Engravings,* Worcester, Mass.,
American Antiquarian Society, 1952.

R. Butterfield, *The American Past,* New York, New York,
Simon and Schuster, 1947.

S. G. L. Dannett, *A Treasury of Civil War Humor,* New York,
New York, Thomas Yoseloff, 1963.

C. W. Dreppard, *Early American Prints,* New York, New York,
The Century Co., 1930.

Charles Evans, *American Bibliography,* Vol. 4, Chicago, Ill.,
Blakely Press, 1907.

Foreign Policy Association, *A Cartoon History of the
United States Foreign Policy 1776-1976,* New York, New York,
Wm. Morrow and Co., 1975.

F. H. Garrison, *An Introduction to the History of Medicine,*
ed. 3, Philadelphia, Pennsylvania, W. B. Saunders Co., 1924.

M. D. George, *English Political Caricature,* 2 vols.,
Oxford, England, Oxford University Press, 1959.

W. H. Helfand, *Pharmaceutical Themes on Patriotic Envelopes,*
J. Amer. Phar. Assn., N S *10, (7),* 418, 1970.

S. Hess and M. Kaplan, *The Ungentlemanly Art,* New York,
New York, The MacMillan Co., 1968.

W. Murrell, *A History of American Graphic Humor,* 2 vols.,
New York, New York, The MacMillan Co., 1933.

A. Nevins and F. Weitenkampf, *A Century of Political
Cartoons,* New York, New York, Chas. Scribner's Sons, 1944.

A. B. Paine, *Th. Nast, His Period and His Pictures,*
New York, New York, The MacMillan Co., 1904.

A. Shaw, *Abraham Lincoln. The Year of His Election,*
New York, New York, The Review of Reviews Corp., 1929.

F. G. Stevens and E. Hawkins, *Catalog of Prints and Drawings
in the British Museum,* Vol. 4, London, England,
British Museum, 1883.

R. Tyler, *The Image of America in Caricature & Cartoon,*
Ft. Worth, Texas, Amon Carter Museum of Western Art, 1975.

J. C. Vinson, *Thomas Nast—Political Cartoonist,*
Athens, Georgia, Univ. of Georgia Press, 1967.

F. Weitenkampf, *Political Caricature in the United States,*
New York, New York, The New York Public Library, 1953.

R. R. Wilson, *Lincoln in Caricature,* New York, New York,
Horizon Press, 1945.

acknowledgments

I am particularly indebted to the following persons and
institutions for help in preparing this book:

Cynthia A. Angelidis, Harvard University; Alex Berman,
Univ. of Cincinnati; David L. Cowen, Rutgers University;
Virginia Daiker, Library of Congress; James J. Heslin, N.Y.
Historical Society; Milton Kaplan, Library of Congress;
Kneeland McNulty, Phila. Museum of Art; Harold Merklen,
N.Y. Public Library; James E. Mooney, American
Antiquarian Society; Gerald P. Rodnan, Univ. of Pittsburgh;
Elizabeth E. Roth, N.Y. Public Library; Lillian Tonkin,
Library Company of Philadelphia; Ellen Wells, Cornell
University; Richard Wolfe, Countway Library.

sources of illustrations

American Antiquarian Society: 3, 4, 5, 8, 10, 13, 14, 21, 22, 26, 40,
43, 45, 47, 67, 68, 70, 73, 74, 78, 81, 87, 91, 112, 123

Columbia University Library: 19, 31, 92, 98, 100, 103, 110, 111

Francis A. Countway Library of Medicine: 106

Harvard University (Houghton Library): 69, 88

Harvard University (Weidner Library): 16, 80, 89, 90, 101, 102, 105,
108, 109, 115, 116, 119, 120, 122, 124

Historical Society of Pennsylvania: 38, 39, 61, 62

Library Company of Philadelphia: 6, 7, 23, 66, 79

Library of Congress: 71, 95, 97

New York Historical Society: 9, 24, 25, 44, 65, 76, 82, 118, 125

New York Public Library (Astor, Lenox and Tilden Foundations):
1, 2, 12, 27, 28, 29, 32, 34, 37, 41, 42, 46, 72, 75, 94, 96, 107, 114, 117,
121

Princeton University: 11, 15, 20, 35, 63, 64, 83, 84, 85, 86, 93, 99

Rutgers University: 30, 77

University of Cincinnati: 33, 104

The following illustrations are from items in my own collection: 17,
18, 36, 48, 49, 50, 51, 52, 53, 54, 55, 56, 57, 58, 59, 60, 113.

William H. Helfand is a collector of prints relating to medicine and pharmacy and is the author of more than thirty publications on these subjects. He is a past President and Executive Secretary of the American Institute of the History of Pharmacy, and received the Edward Kremers Award for distinguished pharmaco-historical writing from the Institute in 1972.